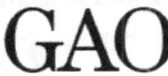

United States Government Accountability Office

Report to Congressional Requesters

I0426228

July 2012

SUPPLEMENTAL NUTRITION ASSISTANCE PROGRAM

Improved Oversight of State Eligibility Expansions Needed

> This report was reissued on August 2, 2012 to add an additional addressee.

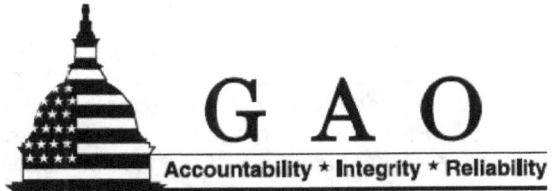

GAO-12-670

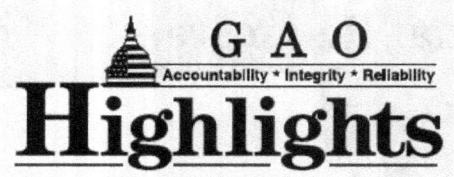

GAO
Accountability * Integrity * Reliability

Highlights

Highlights of GAO-12-670, a report to congressional requesters

SUPPLEMENTAL NUTRITION ASSISTANCE PROGRAM

Improved Oversight of State Eligibility Expansions Needed

Why GAO Did This Study

Over the last 10 years, participation in the U.S. Department of Agriculture's (USDA) SNAP, previously known as the Food Stamp Program, has more than doubled, and costs have quadrupled. Since 1999, USDA has allowed states to expand SNAP eligibility by adopting BBCE policies, which make households that receive services funded by Temporary Assistance for Needy Families, such as a toll-free number or brochure, categorically eligible for SNAP. Under BBCE policies, states are able to increase federal SNAP limits on household income and remove limits on assets. Although USDA has encouraged states to adopt BBCE to improve SNAP access and administration, little is known about the effects of these policies. GAO was asked to assess: (1) To what extent are households that would otherwise be ineligible for SNAP deemed eligible for the program under BBCE? (2) What effect has BBCE had on program costs? (3) What are the program integrity implications of BBCE? GAO analyzed data from USDA, selected states, and other national sources; conducted site visits to 5 states; and interviewed federal, state, and local officials, as well as others with knowledge of SNAP.

What GAO Recommends

GAO recommends that USDA review state procedures for implementing BBCE, disseminate guidance to states on certifying SNAP households as eligible for school meals, and revisit its guidance on SNAP reporting requirements to ensure they address all households. USDA generally agreed with GAO's recommendations.

View GAO-12-670. For more information, contact Kay Brown at (202) 512-7215 or brownke@gao.gov.

What GAO Found

In fiscal year 2010, GAO estimates that 2.6 percent (473,000) of households that received Supplemental Nutrition Assistance Program (SNAP) benefits would not have been eligible for the program without broad-based categorical eligibility (BBCE) because their incomes were over the federal SNAP eligibility limits. The characteristics of these households were generally similar to other SNAP households, although they were more likely to work or receive unemployment benefits. BBCE removes asset limits in most states, and while reliable data on participants' assets are not available, other data suggest few likely had assets over these limits. Although BBCE contributed to recent increases in SNAP participation, other factors, notably the recent recession, had a greater effect.

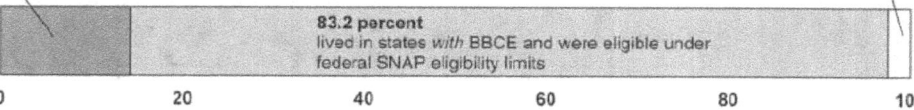

Estimated Sub-groups of SNAP Households, Fiscal Year 2010

14.3 percent lived in states *without* BBCE and were eligible under federal SNAP eligibility limits

2.6 percent lived in states *with* BBCE and had income over federal SNAP eligibility limits

83.2 percent lived in states *with* BBCE and were eligible under federal SNAP eligibility limits

Percentage of all SNAP households

Source: GAO analysis of SNAP quality control data.

GAO estimates that BBCE increased SNAP benefit costs, which are borne by the federal government, by less than 1 percent in fiscal year 2010. In that year, total SNAP benefits provided to households that, without BBCE, would not have been eligible for the program because their incomes were over the federal SNAP eligibility limits were an estimated $38 million monthly or about $460 million for the year. These households received an estimated average monthly SNAP benefit of $81 compared to $293 for other households. BBCE's effect on SNAP administrative costs, which are shared by the federal and state governments, is unclear, in part because of other recent changes that affect this spending, such as state budget and staffing reductions in the recent recession.

BBCE has potentially had a negative effect on SNAP program integrity. In recent years, the SNAP payment error rate declined to an historic low, but evidence suggests the decline is primarily due to changes other than BBCE. While BBCE may improve administrative efficiency, both national data and discussions with local staff suggest BBCE may also be associated with more errors. In addition, BBCE has led to unintended consequences for SNAP and related programs. For example, in implementing BBCE, some states are designating SNAP applicants as categorically eligible without providing them with the service required to make this determination. Further, likely because they are unaware of recent USDA guidance, some states certify children for free school meals when their households are determined eligible for SNAP, even though they do not receive SNAP benefits—a result more common in states with BBCE. Finally, because of federal guidance on BBCE, rules for reporting changes in household circumstances now differ by household income level and may leave higher-income households without reporting requirements for several months.

_____ United States Government Accountability Office

Contents

Figures

Abbreviations

BBCE	broad-based categorical eligibility
FNS	Food and Nutrition Service
SNAP	Supplemental Nutrition Assistance Program
TANF	Temporary Assistance for Needy Families
USDA	U.S. Department of Agriculture

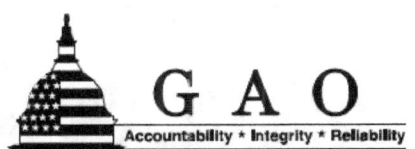

United States Government Accountability Office
Washington, DC 20548

July 26, 2012

The Honorable Frank D. Lucas
Chairman
The Honorable Collin C. Peterson
Ranking Member
Committee on Agriculture
House of Representatives

The Honorable Jeff Sessions
Ranking Member
Committee on the Budget
United States Senate

The Honorable Pat Roberts
Ranking Member
Committee on Agriculture, Nutrition and Forestry
United States Senate

During fiscal year 2011, the U.S. Department of Agriculture's (USDA) Supplemental Nutrition Assistance Program (SNAP), previously known as the Food Stamp Program,[1] provided food and nutrition assistance to almost 45 million individuals each month for a total of $71.8 billion in benefits for the year. SNAP is intended to help low-income individuals and families obtain a better diet by supplementing their incomes with benefits to purchase food. Over the last 10 years, SNAP participation has more than doubled and costs have quadrupled. While some of the recent increases in SNAP participation and costs are due to the recession and benefit increases included in the American Recovery and Reinvestment Act of 2009 (Recovery Act),[2] state policy changes intended to improve program access and simplify the administration of SNAP may also have had an effect.

---

[1]SNAP was given its present name in 2008. Food, Conservation, and Energy Act of 2008, Pub. L. No. 110-346, § 4002(a), 122 Stat. 1651, 1853.

[2]Pub. L. No. 111-5, § 101(a) and (e), 123 Stat. 115, 120.

Under federal law, eligibility for SNAP is based primarily on whether a household's income and assets fall below certain thresholds.[3] In addition, low-income households are categorically eligible for SNAP if they receive benefits from certain other federal programs, such as Temporary Assistance for Needy Families (TANF).[4] Originally, categorical eligibility was designed as a method by which households receiving cash assistance benefits were deemed SNAP-eligible. However, since 1999, USDA has allowed states to expand categorical eligibility to households authorized to receive TANF-funded non-cash services by adopting broad-based categorical eligibility (BBCE) policies.[5] Under BBCE policies, states align the SNAP household income and asset limits in federal law with the income and asset limits for the relevant TANF-funded non-cash service. While SNAP eligibility limits therefore differ among states that have adopted BBCE policies, the amount of assistance eligible households receive is determined using the same process for all SNAP applicants. From fiscal year 2006 through fiscal year 2012, the number of states with BBCE policies increased from 7 to 43.

Although USDA has encouraged states to adopt BBCE to improve SNAP access and simplify administration, little is known about the impact of BBCE on SNAP. As a result, we were asked to assess: (1) To what extent are households that would otherwise be ineligible for SNAP deemed eligible for the program under BBCE? (2) What effect has BBCE had on program costs? (3) What are the program integrity implications, if any, of BBCE?

As criteria for our review, we examined federal laws affecting SNAP, as well as USDA regulations and guidance related to SNAP and specifically to BBCE. To answer our research questions, we collected and analyzed information through several methods. At the federal level, we reviewed USDA's information on states' BBCE policies and interviewed department officials. We also reviewed USDA's data on SNAP households, program

---

[3]7 U.S.C. § 2014(a).

[4]In addition, households in which all members receive Supplemental Security Income (SSI) or benefits from state or local general assistance programs are categorically eligible for SNAP. 7 U.S.C. § 2014(a).

[5]Letter to Regional Administrators–All Regions, "FSP–Categorical Eligibility," signed by the Deputy Administrator of the Food Stamp Program, Food and Nutrition Service, USDA. July 14, 1999.

costs, and error rates for the 50 states; Washington, D.C.; Guam; and the Virgin Islands. We determined that these data were sufficiently reliable for the purposes of this report. Because USDA's data lack information on the assets of SNAP households deemed eligible under BBCE, which is key to understanding the effects of BBCE on participation and benefit costs, we also reviewed additional national data sources that provide information on household assets, such as the Survey of Consumer Finances, and determined that these data were sufficiently reliable for the purposes of this report. While these data sources provide estimates of the average amount of assets owned by households of different income levels, which can therefore be used to approximate the level of assets owned by SNAP households, they do not directly provide estimates of SNAP households' assets. To gather additional background information on the effects of various factors on SNAP participation and costs, we identified and reviewed additional studies on SNAP conducted by USDA and several research organizations that assess programs for low-income populations.

To gather information from state and local SNAP administrators on the effects of BBCE policies, as well as other simultaneous changes to the program, we conducted site visits to 5 states (Arizona, Illinois, North Carolina, South Carolina, and Wisconsin) and 18 local SNAP offices located in both urban and rural areas in those states. We selected these states because they varied in their BBCE adoption dates, characteristics of their BBCE policies, and geographic locations. States selected also had relatively large SNAP caseloads and generally high proportions of their SNAP households deemed eligible under BBCE policies. Within each state, we interviewed state SNAP administrators, as well as local SNAP administrators from three to four local offices. We cannot generalize our findings from the site visits beyond the states and localities we visited. In addition to our site visits, we also interviewed state SNAP administrators in Idaho and Michigan to gather information on the impacts of the asset limits that these states added to their BBCE policies in 2011. To gather other perspectives about the effects of BBCE on SNAP, we also interviewed officials knowledgeable about SNAP from research and advocacy organizations that focus on nutrition assistance policy.

We conducted this performance audit from August 2011 through July 2012 in accordance with generally accepted government auditing standards. Those standards require that we plan and perform the audit to obtain sufficient, appropriate evidence to provide a reasonable basis for our findings and conclusions based on our audit objectives. We believe that the evidence obtained provides a reasonable basis for our findings and conclusions based on our audit objectives. See appendices I and II for additional information on our objectives, scope, and methodology.

Background

SNAP is the largest of the 15 domestic food and nutrition assistance programs overseen by USDA's Food and Nutrition Service (FNS). FNS jointly administers SNAP with the states. FNS pays the full cost of SNAP benefits and pays approximately half of states' administrative costs.[6] FNS is also responsible for promulgating program regulations and ensuring that state officials administer the program in compliance with program rules. States administer the program by determining whether households meet the program's eligibility requirements, calculating monthly benefits for qualified households, and issuing benefits to participants.

Participation and Costs

As shown in figures 1 and 2, SNAP participation and costs generally increased between fiscal years 2001 and 2011, though the most significant increases began in fiscal year 2008.

---

[6]Generally, FNS reimburses states for 50 percent of most types of SNAP administrative costs. However, some types of administrative costs are reimbursed at higher rates, such as some costs related to employment and training services and computer system development. Further, in response to SNAP participation increases during the recent economic downturn, the American Recovery and Reinvestment Act of 2009 and the Department of Defense Appropriations Act, 2010 made $290.5 million and $400 million, respectively, available to states for SNAP administrative costs in fiscal years 2009-2011. Pub. L. No. 111-5, § 101(c), 123 Stat. 115, 120 and Pub. L. No. 111-118, § 1002(a), 123 Stat. 3409, 3468-69.

Figure 1: Average Monthly Number of SNAP Participants per Fiscal Year, in Millions

Average monthly number of SNAP participants (in millions)

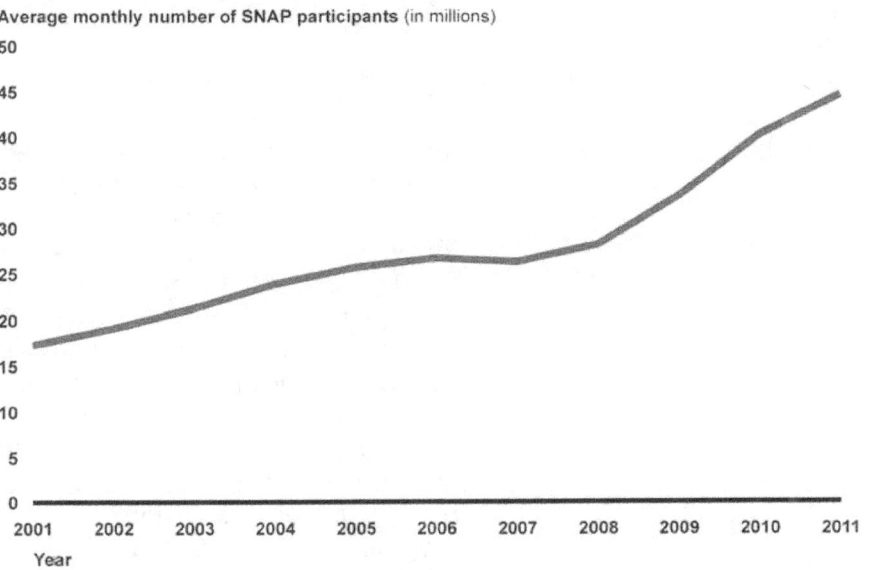

Source: GAO analysis of USDA data on SNAP participants.

Figure 2: Total Federal SNAP Costs per Fiscal Year, in Billions

Total federal SNAP costs (in billions)

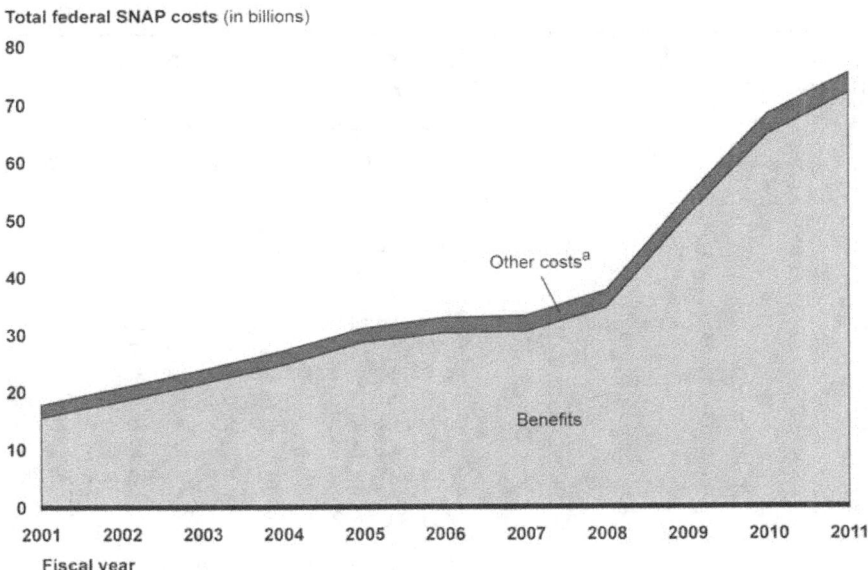

Source: GAO analysis of USDA data on SNAP costs.

Note: "Other Costs" include the federal share of SNAP administrative costs and employment and training programs, as well as other federal costs (e.g., benefit and retailer redemption and monitoring, payment accuracy, electronic benefit transfer systems, program evaluation and modernization, program access, health and nutrition pilot projects).

According to FNS, the growth in SNAP participation in recent years is likely attributable to the economic recession, outreach efforts, and modifications to program policy. Because households must be low-income to receive SNAP benefits, participation and costs typically increase during economic downturns as more people become eligible and apply. Although the recent recession officially lasted from December 2007 through June 2009, since then, unemployment has remained above average levels and SNAP participation has continued to grow. Further, because federal law identifies SNAP's main purpose as "raising levels of nutrition among low-income households,"[7] one of the key performance measures for the program is the rate of participation among eligible households. As a result, for years, FNS has encouraged states to undertake outreach efforts and adopt various modifications to program policy to increase participation among the eligible population and increase program efficiency. Although the participation rate varies by state, ranging from an estimated 53 percent in California to 100 percent in Maine in fiscal year 2009, the national rate has been about 70 percent in recent years.[8]

Determination of Eligibility

Under federal law and regulations, eligibility for SNAP is based primarily on a household's income and assets.[9] A household generally includes everyone who lives together and purchases and prepares meals together.[10] To determine a household's eligibility, a caseworker must first

---

[7] 7 U.S.C. § 2011.

[8] To estimate the program's participation rate, the number of SNAP participants in each state, according to administrative data, is divided by the estimated number of eligible persons. To estimate the number eligible, USDA applies SNAP federal eligibility rules to household data in the U.S. Census Bureau's Current Population Survey. This approach does not take into account households potentially eligible for SNAP in states with BBCE policies that modify the federal eligibility rules. If these households were included, many states' participation rate estimates would likely be lower.

[9] 7 U.S.C. § 2014.

[10] 7 U.S.C. § 2012(n). There are specific exceptions to the definition of a household. For example, husbands, wives, and most children under age 22 that live together are included in the same household, even if they purchase and prepare meals separately.

determine the household's gross income, which cannot exceed 130 percent of the federal poverty guidelines,[11] and its net income, which cannot exceed 100 percent of the guidelines (or $18,530 annually for a family of three living in the continental United States in fiscal year 2012).[12] Net income is determined by taking into account certain exclusions and deductions, for example, expenses for dependent care, utilities, and housing.[13] In addition, a caseworker must determine a household's assets under various requirements. For example, a household's liquid assets, such as those in a bank account, currently cannot exceed $2,000 or, for households with an elderly or disabled member, $3,250.[14] However, certain assets are not counted for SNAP, such as a home, the surrounding lot, and most retirement plans and educational savings accounts.[15] While there are also federal SNAP provisions that limit the value of vehicles an applicant can own and still be eligible for the program,[16] all states have opted to modify those rules, and most exclude the value of all household vehicles. (See figure 3 for a general depiction of the eligibility determination process under federal SNAP rules.)

[11] 7 U.S.C. § 2014(c)(2). The federal poverty guidelines are updated periodically in the *Federal Register* by the Secretary of Health and Human Services. 42 U.S.C. § 9902(2) and (4).

[12] 7 U.S.C. § 2014(c)(1). Households that include an elderly or disabled member do not have to meet the gross income limit but must meet the net income limit. SNAP defines elderly members of a household as those aged 60 and older. 7 U.S.C. § 2012(j)(1).

[13] 7 U.S.C. § 2014(d) and (e). Exclusions include, for example, educational loans, veteran's educational benefits, and income earned by minor children.

[14] 7 U.S.C. § 2014(g)(1).

[15] 7 U.S.C. § 2014(g)(2)–(7).

[16] 7 U.S.C. § 2014(g)(2)(C).

Figure 3: How an Applicant's Eligibility Is Determined under Federal SNAP Guidance

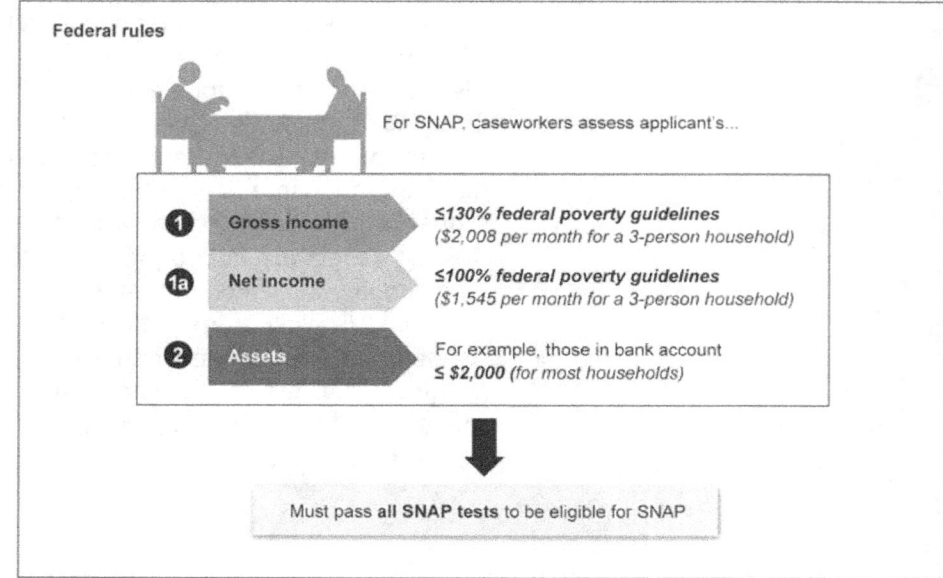

Source: GAO analysis of USDA guidance and SNAP income eligibility standards for fiscal year 2012.

Federal law also allows certain households to be deemed categorically eligible for SNAP.[17] Under statute, households receiving monthly cash assistance from certain programs—including TANF, SSI, and state or local general assistance programs—are categorically eligible for SNAP. According to USDA, categorical eligibility can increase program access and reduce administrative burden, as states assess a household's eligibility once for the cash assistance program rather than twice for both the cash assistance program and SNAP. (See figure 4 for a general depiction of the eligibility determination process under traditional cash assistance-related categorical eligibility.)

---

[17] 7 U.S.C. § 2014(a).

Figure 4: How an Applicant's Eligibility Is Determined under Traditional Cash Assistance-Related Categorical Eligibility

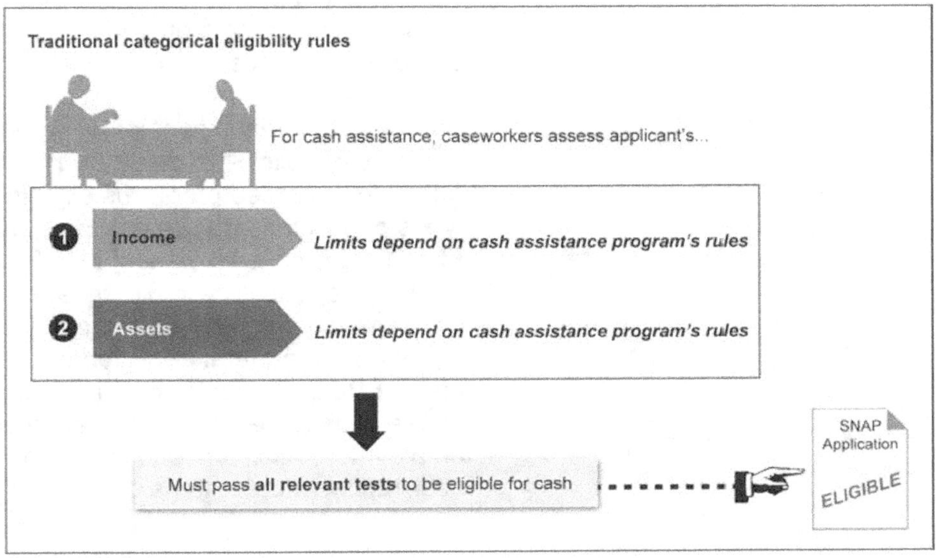

Source. GAO analysis of USDA guidance.

In response to welfare reforms under the Personal Responsibility and Work Opportunity Reconciliation Act of 1996,[18] USDA advised states that households authorized to receive non-cash services—such as case management services, transportation subsidies, or child care subsidies—from a program funded with TANF dollars could also be deemed categorically eligible.[19] In order for a state to fund a non-cash service with TANF dollars, the service generally must further one of TANF's purposes, which include the promotion of job preparation, work, and marriage, and the reduction of out-of-wedlock births.[20] As set out in SNAP regulations, households in which members are authorized to receive non-cash services primarily funded with TANF are categorically eligible, and states also have the option of extending categorical eligibility to households

---

[18]Pub. L. No.104-193, 110 Stat. 2105.

[19]This includes federal TANF dollars and state dollars counted as maintenance-of-effort for TANF. 7 C.F.R. § 273.2(j)(2)(ii) (2012).

[20]42 U.S.C. § 601(a) and 604.

receiving services that are less than 50 percent TANF-funded, with FNS approval required in certain cases.[21] SNAP regulations also direct that the TANF-funded non-cash services used to confer categorical eligibility be available only to households with incomes equal to or below 200 percent of the federal poverty guidelines.

As a result of this expansion of categorical eligibility, states have adopted a variety of policies to deem households that receive non-cash services from TANF-funded programs eligible for SNAP. FNS separates these types of policies into two groups—broad-based and narrow. According to FNS, BBCE policies make most, if not all, households that apply for SNAP categorically eligible because they receive a TANF-funded non-cash service, such as an informational brochure or toll-free number. (See figure 5 for a general depiction of the eligibility determination process under BBCE.) In contrast, narrow categorical eligibility policies require households to be enrolled in certain TANF-funded programs, such as employment assistance, or receiving child care or transportation assistance, in order to be categorically eligible for SNAP.

---

[21] 7 C.F.R. § 273.2(j)(2)(i)-(iii) (2012).

Figure 5: How an Applicant's Eligibility May Be Determined under BBCE

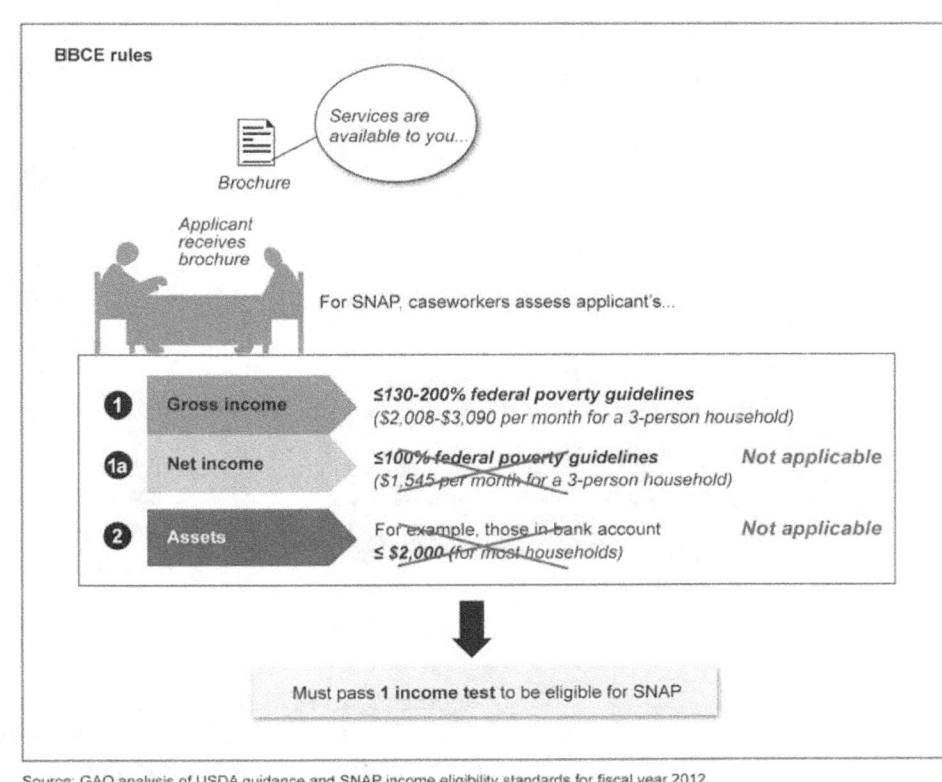

BBCE rules

Services are available to you...

Brochure

Applicant receives brochure

For SNAP, caseworkers assess applicant's...

1	Gross income	≤130-200% federal poverty guidelines ($2,008-$3,090 per month for a 3-person household)	
1a	Net income	~~≤100% federal poverty guidelines ($1,545 per month for a 3-person household)~~	*Not applicable*
2	Assets	~~For example, those in bank account ≤ $2,000 (for most households)~~	*Not applicable*

Must pass **1 income test** to be eligible for SNAP

Source: GAO analysis of USDA guidance and SNAP income eligibility standards for fiscal year 2012.

Note: This figure depicts the general process for determining a household's SNAP eligibility in a state with a BBCE policy that removes the federal SNAP asset limit and does not include a net income limit. Not all states have such a policy.

Although FNS issued guidance in 1999 and regulations in 2000 explaining how states could adopt BBCE policies,[22] relatively few states implemented them early on. Between fiscal years 2001 and 2006, 7 states adopted these policies. However, when the recent economic downturn began, and households applying for SNAP began to increase greatly, FNS encouraged states to adopt these policies to streamline eligibility processes and ease workload (see fig. 6).

---

[22]65 Fed. Reg. 70,134, 70,160 and 70,198 (Nov. 21, 2000). Although promulgated in 2000, none of its provisions became effective prior to January 20, 2001.

Figure 6: Timeline of State BBCE Policy Implementation, Fiscal Years 2001-2012

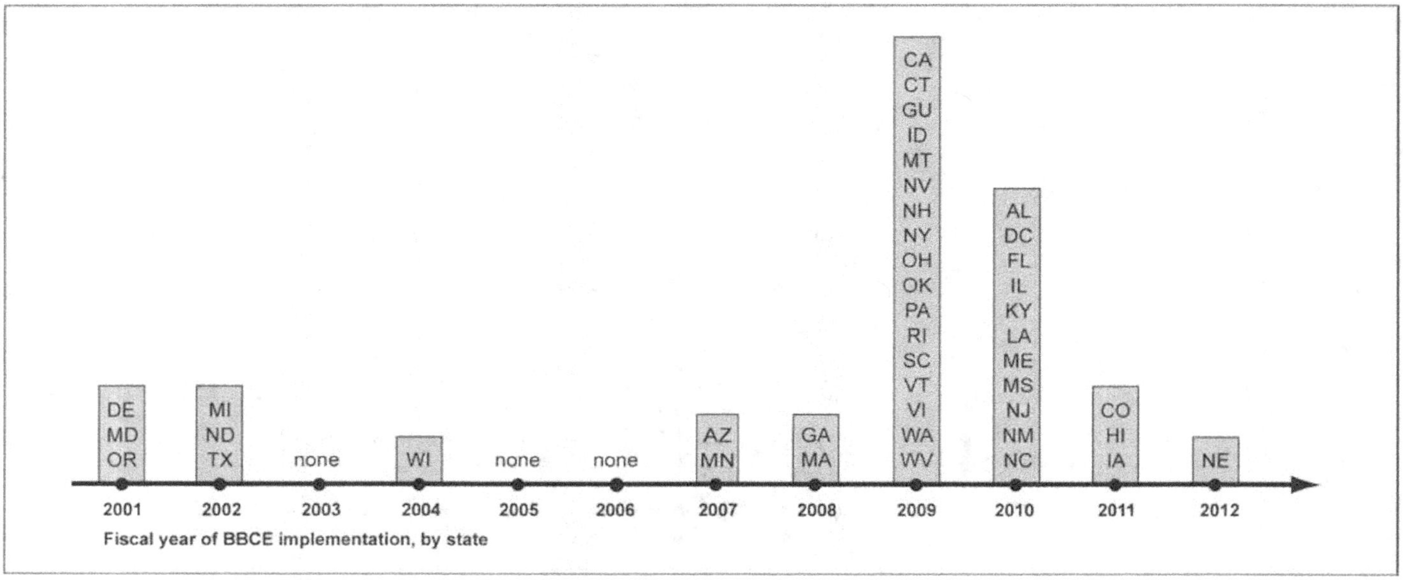

Source: USDA data on state implementation of BBCE policies.

According to FNS, as of May 1, 2012, 43 states—including Washington, D.C., Guam, and the Virgin Islands—had BBCE policies.[23] These policies differ in terms of the income and asset limits used to determine eligibility, as shown in table 1. For example, 24 states' BBCE policies increase the federal gross income limit for SNAP and remove the asset limit while 2 states' BBCE policies retain the federal gross income limit and increase the federal asset limit.

---

[23]For this report, we reviewed information on SNAP in the 50 states; Washington, D.C.; Guam; and the Virgin Islands. We use "states" throughout the report to refer to this group.

Table 1: Number of States with Various Income and Asset Limits for Programs Used to Confer BBCE, as of May 1, 2012

	Higher asset limit than federal SNAP limits	No asset limit
Federal SNAP gross income limit equal to 130 percent of the federal poverty guidelines	2	14[a]
Higher gross income limit (160-200 percent of the federal poverty guidelines)	3	24

Source: GAO analysis of USDA data on states' BBCE policies.

[a]Nine of these states increased the federal gross income limit to 200 percent of the federal poverty guidelines, but only for households with elderly or disabled members.

Determination of Benefits

After eligibility is established, benefits are determined based on each household's monthly net income, with greater benefits provided to those with less income. SNAP expects each eligible household to spend 30 percent of its own resources on food, and therefore, each household's monthly SNAP benefit is determined by subtracting 30 percent of its monthly net income from the maximum SNAP benefit for the relevant household size.[24] All eligible one- and two-person households are guaranteed a minimum benefit, which is $16 for households in the continental United States in fiscal year 2012.[25] However, households with three or more members do not receive a minimum benefit. Under federal income eligibility limits, a household with three or more members will typically be determined eligible for a SNAP benefit greater than $0. However, because some states' BBCE policies raise the SNAP income limits, under these policies, such households are more likely to be deemed eligible for $0 in benefits.

Certification and Reporting Requirements

SNAP households are certified eligible for SNAP for periods ranging from 1 to 24 months, which vary based on state policy choices. Generally, the length of the certification period depends on household circumstances,

[24]7 U.S.C. § 2017(a) If a household has zero net income (that is, its deductable expenses equal or exceed its gross income), it receives the maximum SNAP benefit based on household size. Maximum benefits are based on USDA's Thrifty Food Plan, which is an estimate of how much it costs to buy food to prepare nutritious, low-cost meals for a household. The Thrifty Food Plan estimate is changed every year to keep pace with food prices.

[25]7 U.S.C. § 2017(a). The minimum benefit for eligible one- and two-person households in Alaska, Hawaii, Guam, and the Virgin Islands ranges from $19-$30 in fiscal year 2012.

but only households in which all members are elderly or disabled can be certified for up to 24 months under federal regulations.[26] Once the certification period ends, households reapply for benefits, at which time eligibility and benefit levels are redetermined.

Between certification periods, households generally must report changes in their circumstances—such as household composition, income, and expenses—that may affect their eligibility or benefit amounts.[27] Since early 2001, states have had the option of requiring households to report changes only when their incomes rise above 130 percent of the federal poverty guidelines, rather than reporting changes at regular intervals or within 10 days of occurrence, as was required in the past.[28] According to FNS, as of November 2010, all states except California and Wyoming use this simplified reporting for some or all SNAP households.

Quality Control System

FNS and the states share responsibility for implementing an extensive quality control system used to measure the accuracy of SNAP eligibility and benefits and from which state and national error rates are determined.[29] Under FNS's quality control system, the states calculate their payment errors annually by drawing a statistical sample to determine whether participating households are eligible and received the correct benefit amount. Because SNAP considers many factors in determining each household's benefit amount, any of these factors can result in a payment error. For example, incorrect calculations of earned income or unearned income and inaccurate accounting of the number of household members may cause payment errors. The state's payment error rate is based on the sample and determined by dividing the dollars paid in error by the total SNAP benefits issued. Once the payment error rates are determined, FNS is required to compare each state's performance with

[26]7 C.F.R. § 273.2(f)(1) (2012). The state must have at least one contact with these households every 12 months.

[27]7 C.F.R. § 273.12(a) (2012).

[28]7 C.F.R. § 273.12(a)(1)(vii) (2012) and 65 Fed. Reg. 70,134, 70,143 and 70,208 (Nov. 21, 2000) (effective Jan. 20, 2001).

[29]The SNAP error rate is calculated for the entire program, as well as every state, and is a combination of overpayments to those who are eligible for smaller benefits, overpayments to those who are not eligible for any benefit, and underpayments to those who do not get as much as they should.

the national payment error rate and impose financial penalties or provide financial incentives according to legal specifications.

While State Eligibility Changes Expanded Participation, the Economy Likely Played a Larger Role

More Became Eligible but Impact of Changes Likely Limited

In fiscal year 2010, an estimated 2.6 percent[30] (approximately 473,000) of all households receiving SNAP benefits nationwide would not have been eligible for the program without BBCE because their incomes were greater than the income limits defined in federal law.[31][32] However, over half of the states did not have BBCE policies that increased SNAP income limits above the federal limits in fiscal year 2010. In the 24 states whose BBCE policies raised household income limits above the federal limits in that year, around 4.8 percent of SNAP households had incomes over those limits (see fig. 7). Those households eligible solely because of BBCE generally had incomes that were modestly higher than the federal limits. On average, their total monthly income was an estimated $1,965,

---

[30]The 95 percent confidence interval for the 2.6 percent estimate is (2.4, 2.8). For the 95 percent confidence intervals for all estimates in this paragraph, see appendix II, table 4.

[31]For more information about our analysis, see appendix I. As previously noted, household eligibility is determined by local staff administering SNAP, and the accuracy of those determinations is assessed by state and federal reviewers. We did not independently determine households' eligibility.

[32]In April 2012, the Congressional Budget Office (CBO) released a report on SNAP that estimates a 4.3 percent annual reduction in SNAP participants over the 2013-2022 period if federal SNAP income and asset limits were applied to all categorically eligible households. However, CBO's methodology for producing its estimates differs from our methodology in several ways. For example, although CBO indicates its estimates reflect changes to BBCE, the Office's estimates include both participants deemed eligible under BBCE policies, as well as those deemed eligible under narrow non-cash categorical eligibility policies. In addition, CBO estimates include assumptions about the share of these households that exceed federal asset limits.

which is about 150 percent of the federal poverty guidelines,[33] whereas the federal income limit for SNAP is 130 percent of the guidelines.

Figure 7: SNAP Households That Would Not Have Been Eligible for the Program without BBCE because Their Incomes Were over Federal Limits, in Fiscal Year 2010

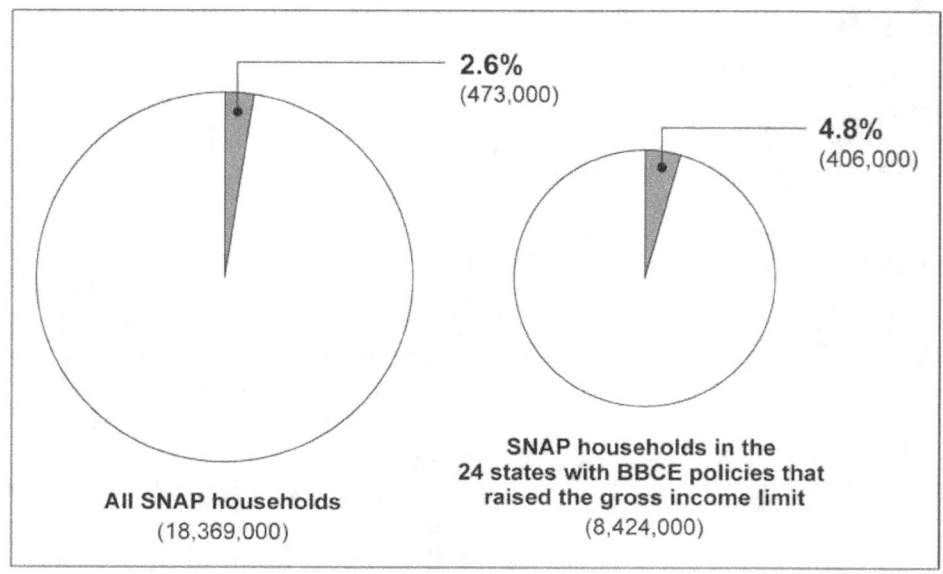

Source: GAO analysis of USDA's SNAP quality control data.

Note: For the 95 percent confidence intervals for these estimates, see appendix II, table 4.

Households eligible under BBCE with incomes over the federal limits had characteristics that were generally similar to all other SNAP households; however, they were more likely to be working or receiving unemployment benefits (see table 2). About half of these households included a child, as was the case for all other SNAP households, and a similar proportion of each group of households included a single female head of household. While a generally similar proportion of both groups of households were elderly recipients of Social Security benefits, the average monthly amount of Social Security benefits received by households that would have failed

---

[33]In fiscal year 2010, 150 percent of the federal poverty guidelines equaled $1,821 monthly for a 2-person household and $2,289 monthly for a 3-person household. We estimate that households with incomes over the federal limits in fiscal year 2010 had, on average, 2.2 members.

the federal income tests was substantially higher. In two of the local offices we visited, staff noted that BBCE may have increased the number of elderly applicants since the policy change enabled some who were previously ineligible because of their Social Security earnings to become eligible for SNAP. Also, although both groups had the same proportion of households with unearned income, a higher percentage of households with incomes above the federal limits had members who worked or who received Unemployment Insurance benefits. Further, the average monthly amount they received in Unemployment Insurance was considerably higher than that received by all other SNAP households.

Table 2: Characteristics of Specified Groups of SNAP Households, in Fiscal Year 2010

	SNAP households with incomes over federal income limits	All other SNAP households
Total number of SNAP households	473,381	17,895,847
Percentage of households with at least one child	56.3	48.5
Percentage of households with a single female as the head	30.7	25.8
Percentage of households with at least one member receiving Social Security benefits	27.8	21.2
Average amount of Social Security benefits received	$340	$155
Percentage of households with at least one member with unearned income	60.0	60.3
Percentage of households with at least one member with earned income	65.9	29.0
Percentage of households with at least one member receiving Unemployment Insurance benefits	18.6	6.4
Average amount of Unemployment Insurance benefits received	$223	$55

Source: GAO analysis of USDA's SNAP quality control data.

Note: The average amount of Social Security and Unemployment Insurance benefits received was calculated for all households in each group, rather than only for households that received these benefits. For the 95 percent confidence intervals for these estimates, see appendix II, table 5.

Available data suggest few households that qualified for SNAP under BBCE likely had assets that would have exceeded federal asset limits. In fiscal year 2010, 37 states had removed the federal asset limit, which was $2,000 for most households,[34] as part of their BBCE policies. Because asset information was therefore not collected from SNAP applicants in these states, USDA's data on SNAP households cannot be used to estimate the number or share of participating households with assets over the federal limits. However, other national data sources suggest the number is relatively small. For example, a national survey that gathered information on families' assets in 2010 found that an estimated 24 percent of families in the bottom income quintile did not have a checking, savings, or other financial transaction account.[35] Among the estimated 76 percent of this group that had such an account, the median balance was an estimated $700. This survey also found that while a greater proportion of families in the second lowest income quintile had such an account in 2010 (91 percent), their median account balance was an estimated $1,500. For the most part, SNAP households deemed eligible under BBCE—households with incomes under 200 percent of the federal poverty guidelines—fall within the two lowest income quintiles.[36] A 2007 survey of families with children found that those with incomes between 100 and 199 percent of the federal poverty guidelines held median liquid assets of around $300.[37] For those with incomes below 100 percent of the guidelines, the median amount was estimated to be zero.

Available state-level data, as well as information shared by state and local officials during our site visits, also suggest the value of assets held by

---

[34]As previously noted, federal SNAP asset limits are $2,000 for most households and $3,250 for households with an elderly or disabled member.

[35]Federal Reserve Board, 2010 Survey of Consumer Finances. Transaction accounts include checking, savings, and money market deposit accounts; money market mutual funds, and call or cash accounts at brokerages.

[36]According to U.S. Census Current Population Survey data, as of March 2010, families with incomes of an estimated $27,379 or less were in the bottom income quintile, and those with estimated incomes from $27,380 to $48,705 were in the second lowest income quintile, in 2010 dollars.

[37]University of Michigan, Institute for Social Research, 2007 Panel Study of Income Dynamics. In this survey, liquid assets are defined as immediately available assets that can be easily converted to cash. These include, for example, the value of checking and savings accounts, as well as stocks, bonds, and cash-value of life insurance. Further, note that families with no liquid assets are included in this analysis.

SNAP households is low. For example, according to state officials in Idaho and Michigan, both states initially removed the federal asset limits as part of their BBCE policies but reinstated an asset limit of $5,000 during 2011. Officials indicated that the new limits had a very small impact on overall caseloads. For example, during the 9 months following Idaho's reinstatement, approximately 850 new applicants and existing recipients seeking recertification were denied benefits because their assets exceeded the asset limit. This represented less than a 1 percent reduction in the total number of SNAP households in that state during that period.[38] Similarly, during the month following Michigan's reinstatement of the asset limit, about 1 percent of the state's existing SNAP cases were closed due to assets.[39] Further, during our site visits, caseworkers in all of the offices we visited said they believe the value of assets held by SNAP households is usually very low or $0. Several caseworkers said that while they may have served SNAP applicants that held assets greater than the federal limits, they believe such instances are rare. Many caseworkers noted it is common to hear from applicants that they have exhausted a significant portion of their available assets before applying for SNAP.

Economic Downturn a Major Cause of Recent Trends

While implementation of BBCE by many states has enabled more households to receive SNAP, the nation's recent economic downturn has likely played a larger role in the increases in participation during the past decade. As shown in figure 8, increases and decreases in SNAP participation often coincide with similar changes in unemployment and poverty. A 2002 USDA study found that during past economic recessions, a 1 percentage-point increase in the national unemployment rate has been associated with an increase in the number of SNAP participants of 1

---

[38]For the 9 full months after reinstatement, the average monthly SNAP caseload in Idaho was approximately 101,000 households.

[39]However, according to Michigan officials, this figure includes both cases closed because they had assets over the $5,000 limit, as well as those closed because they had vehicles worth more than the $15,000 limit that the state simultaneously established. Also, since both Idaho and Michigan's new $5,000 asset limits are higher than the federal SNAP asset limits, it is likely that these estimates are lower than they would be if the states had reinstated the federal asset limits.

GAO-12-670 Supplemental Nutrition Assistance Program

to 3 million.[40] This relationship also existed during the most recent economic recession of 2007-2009,[41] which was marked by a steep rise in the nation's unemployment rate and an increase in the proportion of families living in poverty. Between fiscal years 2007 and 2010, the number of SNAP participants rose by around 14 million (or approximately 54 percent), while the unemployment rate increased by 5 percentage points. This relationship was also noted by staff administering SNAP in all 18 local offices we visited who cited the economic downturn, and related unemployment, as the primary cause of the increases in SNAP participation in their localities.

---

[40]Kenneth Hanson and Craig Gunderson, *How Unemployment Affects the Food Stamp Program,* USDA Economic Research Service, FANRR-26-7 (Washington, D.C.: September 2002). GAO and others have also noted the relationship between unemployment and SNAP. See GAO, *Domestic Food Assistance: Complex System Benefits Millions, but Additional Efforts Could Address Potential Inefficiency and Overlap among Smaller Programs,* GAO-10-346 (Washington, D.C.: April 15, 2010); and James Mabli and Carolina Ferrerosa, *Supplemental Nutrition Assistance Program Caseload Trends and Changes in Measures of Unemployment, Labor Underutilization, and Program Policy from 2000 to 2008* (Cambridge, MA: Mathematica Policy Research, Inc., October 18, 2010).

[41]According to the National Bureau of Economic Research, the U.S. economy was in recession from December 2007 to June 2009.

Figure 8: Trends in SNAP Participation, Unemployment, and Poverty, 1990-2011

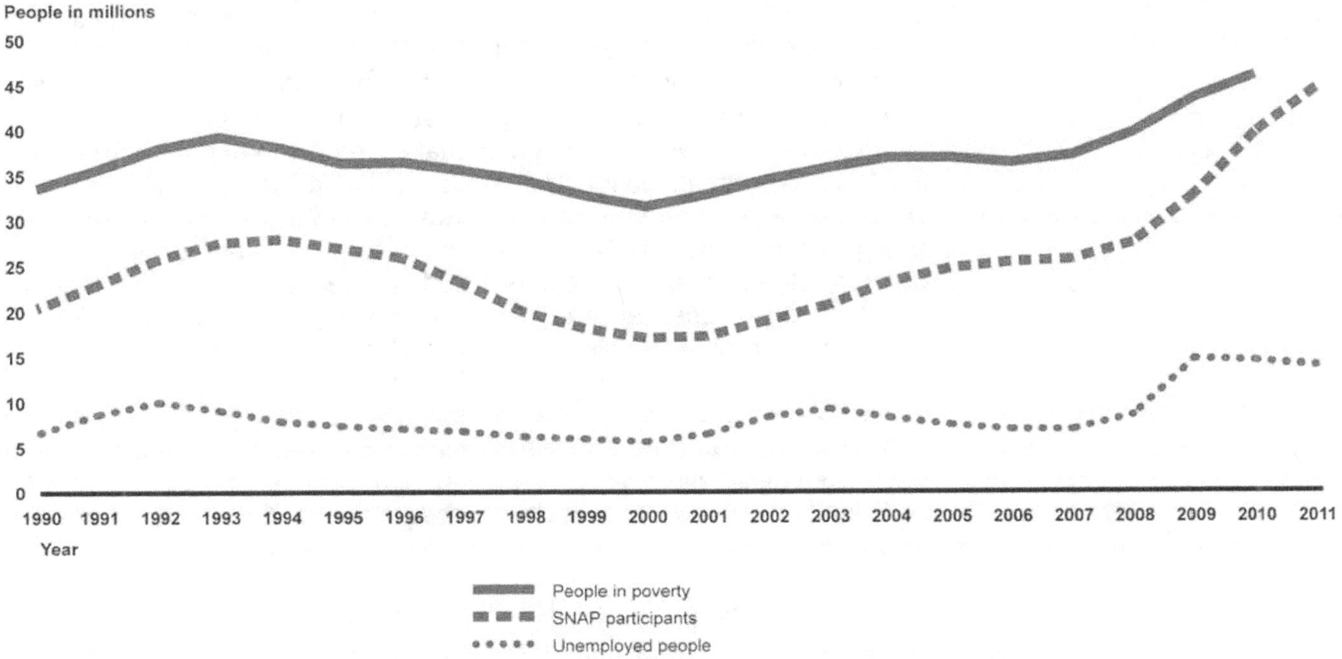

People in millions

	People in poverty
	SNAP participants
	Unemployed people

Source: U.S. Census data on people in poverty, USDA data on SNAP participants, and Bureau of Labor Statistics data on unemployed people.

Note: Numbers of people in poverty are based on data for March of the following year (except the 2010 figure is based on June 2010 data). Numbers of SNAP participants are based on the average monthly value for the fiscal year. Unemployed people are based on data as of June of that year.

Federal changes to SNAP, as well as those initiated by individual states, and a shift in public perception of the program, have also likely contributed to increases in participation during the past decade. For example, the Recovery Act implemented a 13.6 percent increase in maximum monthly SNAP benefits,[42] which likely made participation in the program more attractive to eligible households. In addition, the simplified reporting option, which most states have implemented since it became available in 2001, has been linked to increased participation, likely because it reduces the administrative burden for SNAP households and lengthens certification periods. Further, USDA expenditures targeted to

---

[42]§ 101(a), 123 Stat. 120.

state and community outreach efforts, as well as relaxed limits on vehicle ownership, have been linked to increased SNAP participation. During our site visits, officials noted that the Recovery Act's suspension of the 3-month time limit for able-bodied adults without dependents also caused a noticeable increase in SNAP participants.[43] In addition, individual states have implemented program changes that may have increased participation, such as taking steps to make it easier to apply for SNAP. For example, staff in most of the states we visited cited implementation of online applications and phone interviews, instead of in-person interviews, as improving access to SNAP and shifting the public's perception of the program. Some local caseworkers noted that being able to apply without going to a public assistance office lowers the stigma associated with receipt of government assistance. These changes may also be encouraging participation among specific age groups, as local caseworkers across several states we visited described an increasing trend of single people aged 22 applying as their own SNAP households.[44] Several studies have examined the impact of various changes on SNAP participation, though it is difficult to measure the precise impact of any single change.[45]

Other studies, our own analysis of USDA data, and information we obtained during our site visits indicate the impact of BBCE on SNAP participation is likely small, and the extent to which the policy directly encouraged eligible households to participate is uncertain. While several studies have concluded that BBCE policies have contributed to increases

[43]§ 101(e), 123 Stat. 121. The Recovery Act eliminated the SNAP time limit for these adults without dependents during the period April 1, 2009, through September 30, 2010, but most states have since received waivers to continue the time limit suspension through fiscal year 2013.

[44]At age 22, a SNAP applicant can be declared a separate household, even if living with friends or family. 7 C.F.R. § 273.1(b)(ii). Caseworkers noted that they have seen some people apply for SNAP on their 22nd birthdays, and they believe that online information about program rules, as well as online applications, may be affecting this trend.

[45]Caroline Ratcliffe, Signe-Mary McKernan, and Kenneth Finegold, *The Effect of State Food Stamp and TANF Policies on Food Stamp Program Participation* (Washington, D.C.: The Urban Institute, March 2007); James Mabli, Emily Sama Martin, and Laura Castner, *Effects of Economic Conditions and Program Policy on State Food Stamp Program Caseloads, 2000 to 2006* (Washington, D.C.: Mathematica Policy Research, Inc., August 2009); and Jacob Alex Klerman and Caroline Danielson, *Determinants of the Food Stamp Program Caseload* (Washington, D.C.: RAND, January 2009).

in SNAP participation,[46] they yield inconclusive results concerning the magnitude of the impact. Our own analysis of changes in SNAP participation in the 17 states that adopted BBCE policies during fiscal year 2009 revealed those states had a slightly larger increase in participation between fiscal years 2008 and 2010 than states without BBCE. However, because of the many other factors influencing SNAP participation during these years, we cannot attribute this increase entirely to BBCE. State officials and local caseworkers in the five states we visited were also uncertain of BBCE's effect on SNAP participation. According to those we spoke to, BBCE had a noticeable, but relatively small, effect on SNAP participation, and local staff in all 18 of the offices we visited said BBCE's impact on SNAP participation was considerably less than that caused by the economic downturn. Those in one office said they had been alerted by their state office to prepare for a significant spike in applications once the BBCE policy went into effect, but the subsequent increase was considerably less than expected. Others noted that the participation increases they noticed after BBCE implementation may also have been due to some other simultaneous cause, such as seasonal increases.

---

[46] Jacob Alex Klerman and Caroline Danielson, "The Transformation of the Supplemental Nutrition Assistance Program," *Journal of Policy Analysis and Management*, vol. 30, no. 4, (2011); Janna Johnson, *The Dynamics of SNAP Participation and the Increase in SNAP Caseloads during the Recovery of 2003-2007* (Madison, WI: Institute for Research on Poverty, November 30, 2011); Mabli, Martin, and Castner, *Effects of Economic Conditions and Program Policy on State Food Stamp Caseloads, 2000 to 2006*; and Ratcliffe, McKernan, and Finegold, *The Effect of State Food Stamp and TANF Policies on Food Stamp Program Participation*.

State Eligibility Changes Increased Benefit Costs Somewhat, but Their Effect on Administrative Costs Is Unclear

Benefit Costs Increased Less Than 1 Percent

Although SNAP households that had incomes over the federal limits made up an estimated 2.6 percent of the SNAP caseload in fiscal year 2010, this group received an estimated 0.7 percent[47] of all SNAP benefits. These benefits totaled an estimated $38.3 million a month, or approximately $460 million annually.[48] In the group of states that increased the federal SNAP gross income limit with their BBCE policies, benefits provided to households that had incomes over the federal limits were an estimated 1.5 percent of all SNAP benefits (see fig. 9). Due to data limitations, these estimates represent minimums, as they do not include benefits provided to SNAP households deemed eligible under BBCE with assets over the federal SNAP asset limits.[49]

---

[47]The 95 percent confidence interval for the 0.7 percent estimate is (0.6, 0.8). For the 95 percent confidence intervals for all estimates in this paragraph, see appendix II, tables 4 and 6. For more information about our analysis, see appendix I.

[48]In April 2012, CBO released a report on SNAP that estimates $1.2 billion as the average annual savings in spending over the 2013-2022 period if federal SNAP income and asset limits were applied to all categorically eligible households. CBO considers this estimate to be equivalent to a 1.6 percent annual savings for SNAP. However, CBO's methodology for producing its estimates differs from our methodology in several ways. For example, although CBO indicates its estimates reflect changes to BBCE, the Office's estimates include both benefits provided to households deemed eligible under BBCE policies, as well as benefits provided to households deemed eligible under narrow non-cash categorical eligibility policies. In addition, CBO estimates include assumptions about the share of these households that exceed federal asset limits and the benefits they receive.

[49]The national SNAP household data that we used for our analysis does not include reliable information on assets owned by households deemed eligible under BBCE. As a result, our estimates represent minimums that do not include benefits provided to households who had assets over the federal SNAP asset limits.

Figure 9: Benefits Provided to SNAP Households That Would Not Have Been Eligible for the Program without BBCE because Their Incomes Were over Federal Limits, per Month in Fiscal Year 2010

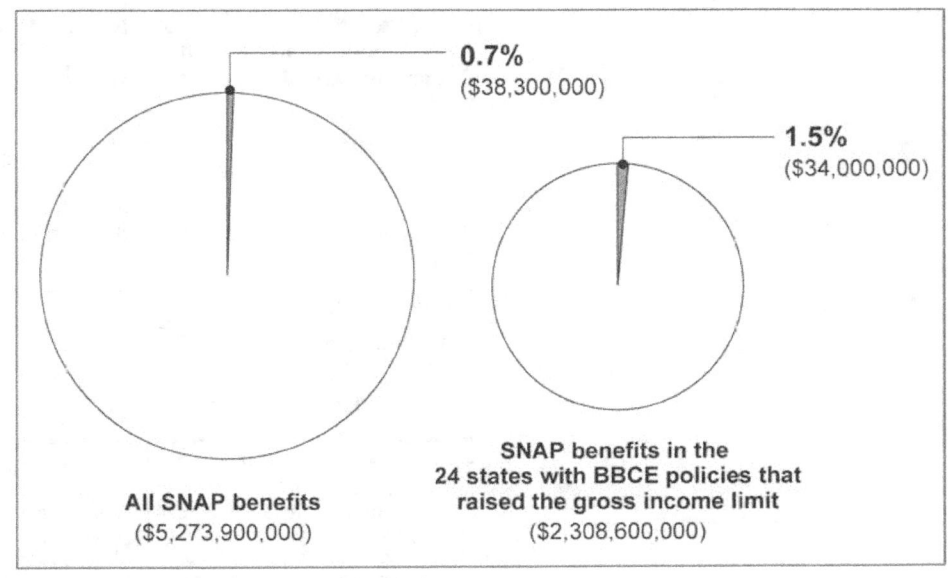

0.7%
($38,300,000)

1.5%
($34,000,000)

All SNAP benefits
($5,273,900,000)

SNAP benefits in the
24 states with BBCE policies that
raised the gross income limit
($2,308,600,000)

Source: GAO analysis of USDA's SNAP quality control data.

Note: For the 95 percent confidence intervals for these estimates, see appendix II, table 6.

Because SNAP benefits are calculated based on income and expenses, and provide greater benefits to those with fewer means, those with incomes over the federal limits tend to be eligible for fewer benefits. On average, these households received an estimated $81 average monthly SNAP benefit in fiscal year 2010 compared to an estimated $293 average monthly benefit received by all other SNAP households in that year.[50] These households also disproportionately received the minimum benefit of $16. An estimated 44 percent of these households received the minimum benefit compared to 3 percent of all other households. Households eligible solely because of BBCE had higher average deductions in certain categories—including dependent care and child support expenses—than other households in fiscal year 2010 (see table 3), and deductions increase monthly SNAP benefits. However, in general,

---

[50]For the 95 percent confidence intervals for all estimates in this paragraph, see appendix II, tables 7 and 8.

　　　　GAO-12-670 Supplemental Nutrition Assistance Program

the higher incomes of households eligible solely because of BBCE seem to have had a greater impact on their SNAP benefits than their deductions, given the relatively low average benefits they received.

Table 3: Estimated Percent of Specified Groups of SNAP Households Receiving Deductions and the Estimated Average Amount of the Deduction, in Fiscal Year 2010

Deduction	Percentage of SNAP households with incomes over the federal limits receiving deduction (average amount)	Percentage of all other SNAP households receiving deduction (average amount)
Child support expenses	6.7 ($20)	1.9 ($4)
Dependent care	14.3 ($50)	3.5 ($8)
Earned income	65.9 ($243)	28.9 ($57)
Medical	13.0 ($19)	3.5 ($5)
Excess shelter	72.2 ($220)	70.5 ($265)

Source: GAO analysis of USDA's SNAP quality control data.

Note: The average amount of the deduction was calculated for all households in each group, rather than only for households that received the deduction. All percentage and numerical estimates in this table are significantly different at the 95 percent confidence level except for the estimated percentage of each group receiving the excess shelter deduction. See appendix II, table 8 for the 95 percent confidence intervals for these estimates.

Both the cost of total SNAP benefits and the average benefit per household increased over the last decade while many states were implementing BBCE; however, other factors likely had a greater effect on benefit costs (see fig. 10). The annual adjustment made to the Thrifty Food Plan—which is the basis for the maximum SNAP benefit amounts, as well as changes in the economy, demographics, and policies affecting deductions, outreach, and eligibility can all affect total spending on SNAP benefits. In recent years, the recession drove increased benefit costs, both by changing household circumstances and by increasing the benefit cost per household. For example, because household benefits are primarily determined based on each household's monthly income, increases in the poverty and unemployment rates likely correlate with increases in the average benefit provided to households. In addition, as previously noted, the Recovery Act implemented a 13.6 percent increase in the maximum monthly SNAP benefit per household. During our site visits, some officials cited these changes as key factors that impacted household benefits in recent years. Officials we spoke to also noted that the slow economic recovery has led to SNAP households remaining on the program for longer time periods than before the recession, which can lead to increases in total benefit costs.

Figure 10: Selected Information on SNAP Benefits and Potentially Related Factors, 2001-2011

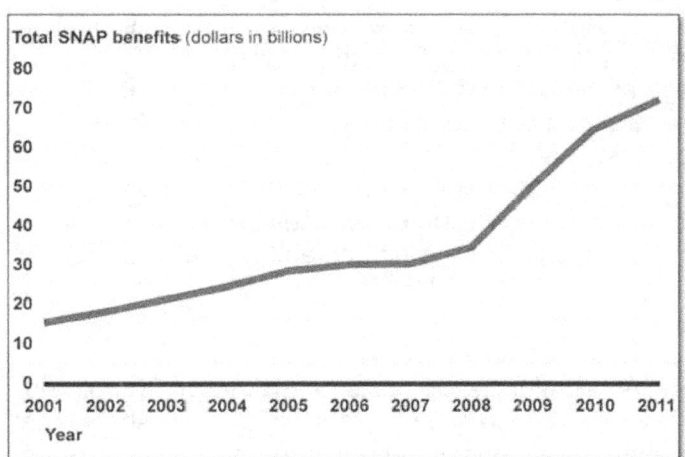

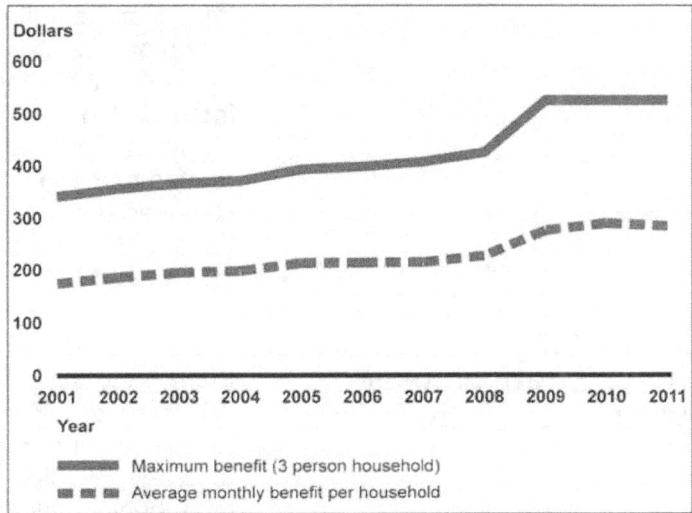

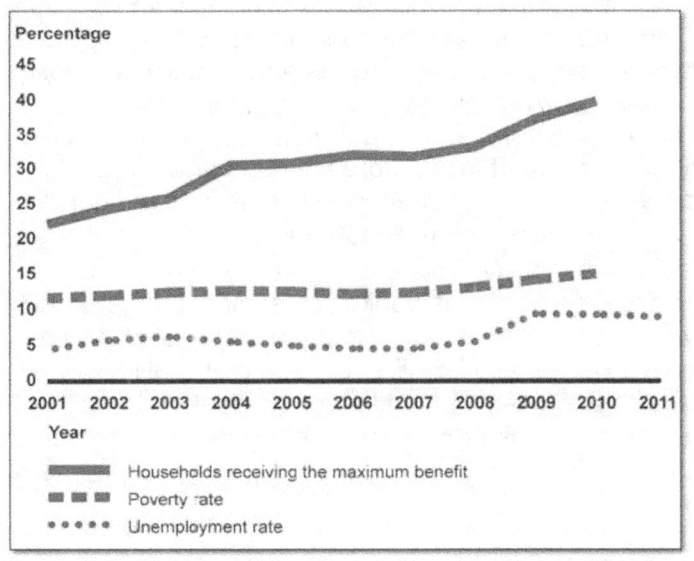

Source: GAO analysis of USDA data on SNAP benefits and households, Bureau of Labor Statistics data on the unemployment rate (in June of each year), and U.S. Census data on the poverty rate.

Because many factors impact SNAP benefit costs, the full extent of BBCE's impact is unclear, though evidence suggests other factors played a more important role in recent years. Although BBCE may impact SNAP benefit costs because the policy both expands who is eligible for the program and streamlines the process for receiving benefits, state and local officials we met with consistently indicated that they did not think

BBCE had a significant impact on benefits. Further, our analysis of SNAP household data suggests factors beyond BBCE typically have a greater impact on benefits. For example, in our review of SNAP benefits in the group of 17 states that implemented BBCE during fiscal year 2009, we found that the average monthly benefit per household significantly increased in all of these states between fiscal years 2008 and 2010. However, for most of these states, the increases were likely primarily related to the increase in maximum benefits implemented under the Recovery Act, as we found no significant differences in the two factors used to determine benefit amounts—net income and household size—for those years.[51]

Administrative Costs Affected by Many Factors

Many factors affect SNAP administrative costs, and state BBCE policies are one factor that may help reduce such costs. Studies have shown that factors ranging from a state's economy and demographic characteristics to its SNAP policies, administrative processes, staff salaries, and the use of technology all impact state administrative spending to varying degrees. As we previously reported, because categorical eligibility policies simplify the eligibility determination process by creating consistency in income and resource limits across programs, these policies can save resources, improve productivity, and help staff focus more time on performing essential program activities.[52] During our site visits, staff in many of the local offices we visited stated that, before BBCE was implemented, verifying assets often took a considerable amount of time, and state officials added that it could be costly, as banks sometimes charge SNAP offices a fee to provide account documentation. As a result, staff in almost all of the local offices we visited said BBCE's removal of the SNAP asset limit helped streamline case processing, and some noted that streamlining occurred both because SNAP households did not have to

---

[51]We found no differences in these two factors in 13 states. However, when comparing SNAP household characteristics for fiscal years 2008 and 2010, we found significant increases in SNAP households' average net income in 3 states that implemented BBCE in fiscal year 2009. In these states, average net income increases appear to be related to higher net incomes in households deemed eligible under BBCE. One state also had a significant decrease in household size.

[52]See GAO, *Human Service Programs: Demonstration Projects Could Identify Ways to Simplify Policies and Facilitate Technology Enhancements to Reduce Administrative Costs*, GAO-06-942 (Washington, D.C.: Sept. 19, 2006).

provide documentation of assets and caseworkers did not need to verify asset information.

Consistent with annual increases in SNAP participation and benefit costs between fiscal years 2001 and 2010, SNAP administrative costs generally increased annually during this period, though at a lower rate. Certification costs—a sub-set of SNAP administrative costs that include the cost of staff determination of household eligibility for benefits—also generally increased over this period (see fig. 11). Cost increases in recent years are likely directly related to the $690.5 million in extra federal funding for SNAP administrative costs provided to states through the Recovery Act and the Department of Defense Appropriations Act, 2010, in response to the national economic recession.[53] However, despite this additional federal funding, because administrative costs increased at a lower rate than SNAP participation, administrative costs per SNAP household declined during this period (see fig. 12).

---

[53]Although the federal government generally funds half of states' administrative costs for SNAP, this additional funding was provided to the states without a requirement that they match it with their own funds.

Figure 11: SNAP Administrative Costs, Fiscal Years 2001-2010

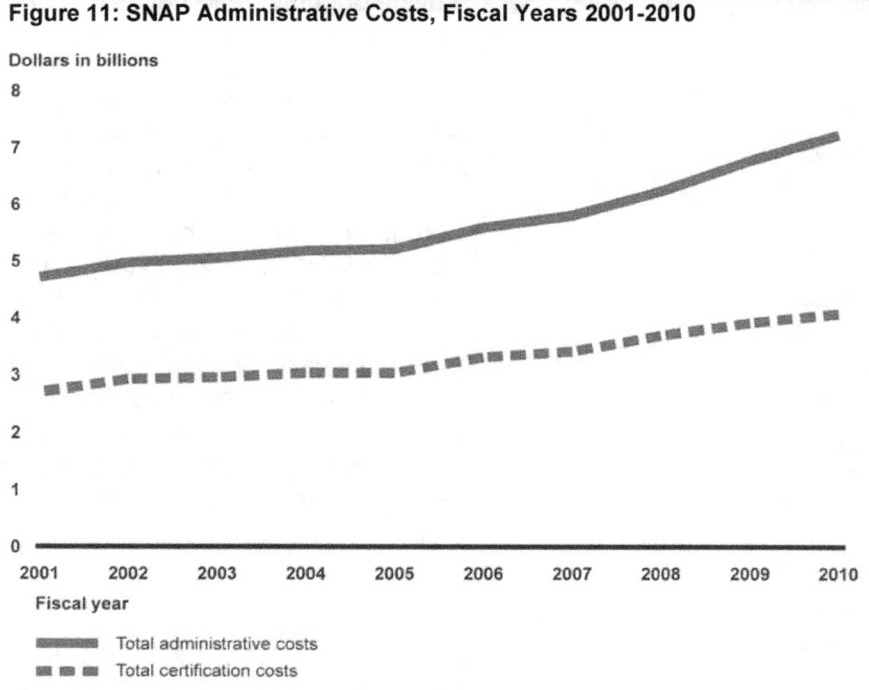

Source: GAO analysis of USDA data on SNAP administrative costs.

Note: These data include administrative costs paid by both federal and state governments.

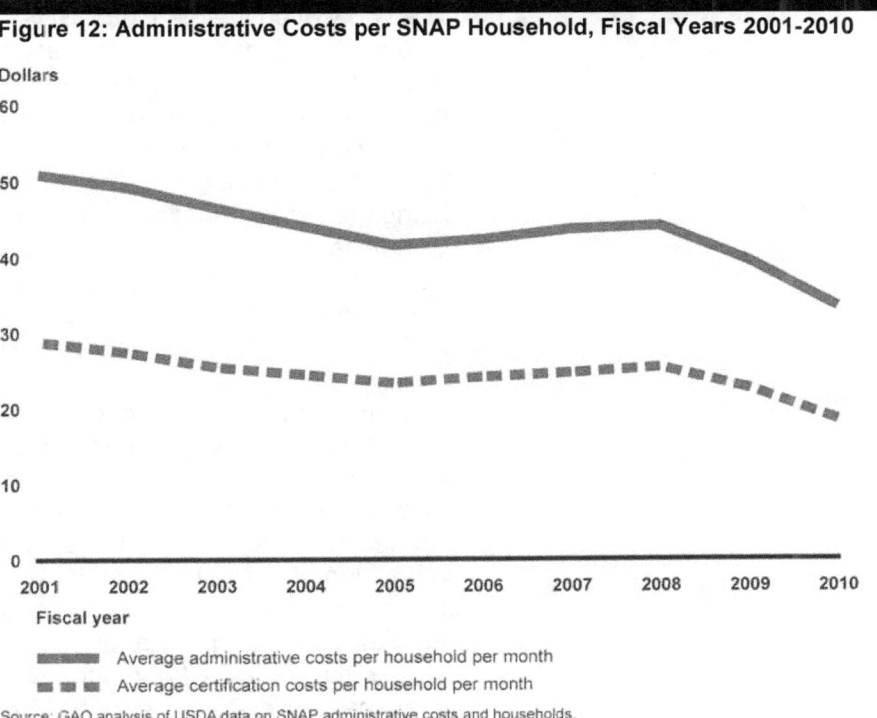

Figure 12: Administrative Costs per SNAP Household, Fiscal Years 2001-2010

——— Average administrative costs per household per month
■ ■ ■ Average certification costs per household per month

Source: GAO analysis of USDA data on SNAP administrative costs and households.

Note: These data include administrative costs paid by both federal and state governments.

While many states implemented BBCE during this period, the largest decreases in these costs occurred in recent years when the economic recession was also a factor. Specifically, during the recent recession, states faced budgetary constraints to funding SNAP administrative expenditures. Because states pay for approximately half of these expenditures, when state tax revenues decrease during recessions, state balanced budget requirements and other constraints affect state and local governments' ability to provide services at the same time that demand for services increases.[54] In our site visits to five states, officials frequently

---

[54]Although the most recent national recession affected states to different degrees, in part depending on their tax structures and economic characteristics, state and local governments generally experienced more severe and long-lasting declines in revenue during this recession when compared to past recessions. For more information on the effect of recessions on state and local governments, see GAO, *State and Local Governments: Knowledge of Past Recessions Can Inform Future Federal Fiscal Assistance,* GAO-11-401 (Washington, D.C.: Mar. 31, 2011).

GAO-12-670 Supplemental Nutrition Assistance Program

noted how overwhelmed local SNAP caseworkers have been with the increased workload during the recent recession. They noted that workload increases have been driven by increases in SNAP participation and the amount of time households remain on the program, as well as budget constraints that hinder their offices' ability to hire additional staff. Across the seven local offices we visited in states that adopted BBCE during the recent recession, staff noted that while BBCE helped streamline the processing of individual cases, these improvements were offset by the increased workload. However, some staff indicated they believe reinstating the federal SNAP asset test that was removed under BBCE would make their workload unmanageable.

In addition to the recession, other changes that states have made to simplify and ease program administration during the last decade make it difficult to determine BBCE's full impact on administrative costs. For example, state and local officials frequently cited the implementation of reduced reporting requirements under the simplified reporting option, the conversion of case files from paper to electronic formats, the implementation of online SNAP applications, and increased use of phone interviews as changes that also helped to ease staff workloads. Officials in one state we visited noted that while these changes may have helped to reduce administrative expenditures over time, some, like BBCE, may have resulted in increased spending in the short-term due to the need for training and modifications to computer systems. Further, while most state SNAP officials we met with during our site visits felt that BBCE likely decreased administrative expenditures to some extent, they did not know the policy's actual impact because of other changes.

State Eligibility Changes May Negatively Affect Program Integrity

Payment Errors May Be Negatively Affected

In recent years, the SNAP payment error rate declined to an historic low while multiple program changes occurred, including BBCE, but evidence suggests that factors other than BBCE may have played a larger role in the decline. Between fiscal years 2000 and 2010, USDA reported that the national payment error rate—the percentage of SNAP benefits paid in error, including underpayments and overpayments—fell from 8.91 percent to 3.81 percent as the number of states with BBCE policies increased from 0 to 39.[55] Because most states' BBCE policies eliminated the need to confirm that SNAP household assets fall below certain limits, BBCE effectively removed the potential for asset-related errors in these states. However, USDA data indicate that most errors have been caused by factors other than assets in recent years. In fact, fewer than 4 percent of all error cases nationally have been caused by asset errors since 2000.[56] Therefore, it is likely that other factors had a greater impact on error rates during this time. For example, the number of states adopting the simplified reporting option for at least some SNAP households increased during this period. Because this option eliminates substantial paperwork requirements for participants and states, and reduces the number of times income is verified, states experience fewer related errors. In addition, states we visited reported that they had also made other changes during this period to help lower their error rates, such as incorporating the use of technology with new case management models or digital files.

Further, both our analysis of USDA data and our discussions with SNAP staff suggest that BBCE may, in fact, contribute to more payment errors. Although BBCE has been promoted by USDA as a possible means to reduce errors, we found that a greater percentage of SNAP households eligible under BBCE that had incomes over the federal limits had payment errors than other households (17.2 percent compared to 6.7 percent) in fiscal year 2010.[57] This may be related to the fact that these households were significantly more likely to have earned income, and income is a frequent cause of SNAP payment errors. In addition, while most states' BBCE policies removed a potential source of error by eliminating asset limits, SNAP caseworkers we spoke with told us that a reduction in the level of verification they perform may actually increase the potential for errors as well as fraud. For example, staff in two states reported that

---

[55]The 95 percent confidence interval for the 8.91 percent estimate is (8.56, 9.26) and the 95 percent confidence interval for the 3.81percent estimate is (3.61, 4.01).

[56]Income-related errors have consistently been the largest contributor to payment errors, representing 49 to 55 percent of all errors since 2000.

[57]The 95 percent confidence interval for the 17.2 percent estimate is (14.3, 20.2), and the 95 percent confidence interval for the 6.7 percent estimate is (6.4, 7.0). These estimates differ from the SNAP payment error rate, as the error rate measures benefit dollars provided in error rather than the percentage of SNAP households with errors.

removing asset verification under BBCE has reduced their ability to investigate other applicant information for possible inconsistencies. Specifically, while asset verification often took considerable time to perform, they noted that previously reviewing bank accounts gave them the ability to identify regular deposits that may be income to ensure those were reported by the applicant. Beyond changes due to BBCE, caseworkers in several states we visited suggested there has been a cultural shift towards an overall reduction in the level of verification and investigation they perform, in part because of the increased participation and workload related to the recent recession. They expressed concern about maintaining a balance between providing assistance to those who need it and ensuring program integrity, noting they worry about losing access to information to help ensure integrity.

Limited Oversight May Contribute to Unintended Consequences

While federal rules provide states with considerable flexibility in designing their BBCE policies, gaps in federal oversight may contribute to some unintended consequences for SNAP and related programs' integrity. We found unintended consequences relating to three key areas:

- provision of a TANF-funded service,[58]
- direct certification for free school meals, and
- requirements for categorically eligible households to report changes (in household circumstances).

TANF-Funded Service Not Consistently Provided

Our visits to states suggest that SNAP applicants are not consistently receiving the TANF-funded information required to confer categorical eligibility and that the extent to which this information is TANF-funded is unclear. According to USDA, BBCE policies make most households that apply for SNAP categorically eligible because they receive a TANF-funded service, such as an informational brochure or toll-free number, as long as the household's income is within the state's specified income limit (see fig. 13).[59] However, in one state we visited, some local SNAP caseworkers told us they did not consistently provide the guide to

---

[58]For this report, we use "TANF-funded service" to refer to a TANF-funded non-cash benefit or service that can be used by states to confer BBCE, per USDA guidance. Per federal regulations, states may grant categorical eligibility to any household authorized to receive a TANF-funded benefit or service. 7 C.F.R. § 273.2(j)(2)(ii) and (iii) (2012).

[59]Applicants may be granted categorical eligibility solely through receipt of such a document, regardless of whether or not they access or receive additional services.

services brochure to all applicants. In another, staff said that at the applicant's request, and/or if caseworkers think there is a need, they will provide referrals to services. In a third state we visited, applicants were directed on the SNAP application to call a toll-free number to receive an informational brochure on services; however, we were unsuccessful in obtaining this brochure after repeated (5) attempts to call the number listed. Further, according to USDA, states must use TANF funds to pay for either the document households receive or the services mentioned in the document. If states use TANF funds to cover at least 50 percent of the cost, they do not need to obtain USDA approval of their BBCE policies. While SNAP officials in three of the states we visited confirmed that the documents used to confer categorical eligibility are partially TANF-funded, they did not know the exact percentage of TANF dollars used to fund them.

Figure 13: Examples of How States Confer BBCE for SNAP

Massachusetts

A Non-Public Assistance food stamp household which consists of adults between the ages of 19 and 59 is subject to the food stamp gross and net income tests and is no longer subject to an asset test. Receipt of the Help for Those in Need: A Resources Brochure confers a TANF Program service.

Nevada

All SNAP applicant households receiving the revised "This is Your Copy" page from the back of the application are categorically eligible for benefits. There will be no resource or gross/net income tests applied to these households. This page was revised to contain the following information about services available from the Nevada Public Health Foundation (NPHF):

Utilizing TANF funds, DWSS through the Nevada Public Health Foundation (NPHF), has developed a class to target pregnant and parenting teens...

Washington

Basic Food Assistance Units with countable income up to 200% of the federal poverty guidelines are eligible to use the department's Online CSO website. This website provides information about our programs as well as referrals to resources in the community. This web-based information and referral service is partly funded with TANF and TANF Maintenance Of Effort funds. Because of this funding, we use this service to make Assistance Units categorically eligible for Basic Food if they have countable income at or under 200%. Clients are notified and authorized to receive this service through a text block on their approval letter for Basic Food.

Source: Commonwealth of Massachusetts, Executive Office of Health and Human Services, Department of Transitional Assistance, Field Operations Memo 2008-27, "Maximized Categorical Eligibility for NPA Food Stamp Households," (May 30, 2008); State of Nevada, Department of Human Resources, Welfare Division, Policy Transmittal, "SNAP Categorical Eligibility – Receipt of TANF Benefit" (March 9, 2009); and Washington State Department of Social and Health Services, Eligibility A-Z Manual, "Categorical Eligibility for Basic Food," (revised February 28, 2012).

Note: We did not conduct site visits to these 3 states, and we did not conduct an independent legal analysis to verify this information.

Gaps in USDA's oversight of states' procedures for implementing BBCE may contribute to the inconsistencies we found in providing qualified applicants with the TANF-funded information or service that confers BBCE. While USDA has issued guidance over the past 3 years in response to various state questions about BBCE, the agency's documentation requirements for states that adopt it are limited. According to agency guidance, while states must document that a household was determined categorically eligible, USDA does not require states to document that the TANF-funded service was received by applicants. As a result, in a state where a document, such as a brochure, is used to confer eligibility, the state does not have to verify that it has provided the document to applicants as part of the eligibility determination process. In addition, headquarters and regional USDA officials told us the agency does not request documentation from states on the extent of TANF funding used, even though that information is necessary to determine whether a BBCE policy would require agency approval. Agency officials added that the burden is on the states to let USDA know if approval is needed. Agency officials also told us that while they provide technical assistance to states, as needed, on the development of their BBCE policies and collect summary information on states' BBCE provisions, they do not approve state BBCE policies.

Inappropriate Certification for Free School Meals

Because states have flexibility to decide how to treat SNAP households deemed eligible for $0 in benefits—an outcome more likely under BBCE—some children have been inappropriately certified for free school meals, including in two states we visited. Under SNAP, states have been allowed to decide whether to deny eligibility to households who qualify for $0 in benefits or whether to certify these households SNAP-eligible without benefits. For school meals programs, statute indicates states must certify children in households that receive SNAP benefits eligible for free school meals—a process called direct certification that is designed to ease administrative burden when certifying children for multiple assistance programs with similar eligibility criteria.[60] Many states rely on data matches between their SNAP program and district-level school data

---

[60]42 U.S.C. § 1758(b)(4). School districts have been required to directly certify SNAP recipients since school year 2008-2009. According to USDA, once a child is directly certified for free school meals, eligibility lasts the entire school year regardless of a change in family circumstances. Households may voluntarily report a change in family circumstances; however, because of the year-long duration of eligibility, households are not required to report changes in their categorical eligibility status.

GAO-12-670 Supplemental Nutrition Assistance Program

to identify children eligible for direct certification, and beginning in school year 2012-2013, all states are expected to do so. However, because a state can certify families receiving $0 in SNAP benefits as eligible in its SNAP data system, it can directly certify children in such families for free school meals, even though they do not receive SNAP benefits.[61] This practice occurred in two states we visited. SNAP officials in one state told us the state adopted BBCE, in part, to potentially enable more children to become eligible for free school meals. Local caseworkers in that state similarly said that they believe parents apply for SNAP specifically because they know their child(ren) are eligible for free school lunch even if they are deemed eligible for $0 in SNAP benefits.

In recognition of this practice, in 2011, USDA issued guidance for states through its regional offices reiterating that children in households receiving $0 in benefits are not categorically eligible for free school meals and therefore should not be directly certified; however, officials in the states we visited were unaware of this guidance. In its October 2011 memorandum, USDA further suggested that state SNAP agencies work with their school meal agency counterparts to ensure that children from $0 benefit SNAP households are excluded from direct certification as soon as possible. According to USDA, school meal agencies were to be in compliance with this guidance by July 1, 2012.[62] Agency officials in USDA's regional offices representing the states we visited told us they routinely transmit guidance and policy changes to states from the national office. This guidance was also made available on USDA's Web site. However, in June 2012, we followed up with the two states we visited that had been directly certifying children from $0 benefit SNAP households, and state officials indicated the practice was still occurring, as they were not aware of this guidance from USDA.

---

[61] This may also impact other programs. For example, some school districts that receive federal funds under Title I, Part A of the Elementary and Secondary Education Act of 1965 (20 U.S.C. § 6301-6339) use the number of children eligible for free and reduced-price meals in each of their schools as a proxy measure of school poverty in order to appropriately distribute those funds to their schools.

[62] Letter to Program Directors-All Regions, "National School Lunch Program and Direct Certification with SNAP," signed by the Director of the Program Development Division, FNS, USDA. October 25, 2011. The practical result is that direct certification of students from families eligible for SNAP but entitled to $0 benefit should not continue in the 2012-13 school year.

Direct certification of children in categorically eligible SNAP households creates another unintended consequence—one of effectively increasing the income eligibility limit for free school meals for some children. While the federal gross income-eligibility limit for SNAP aligns with that of the school meals programs—providing free meal benefits to children in households at or below 130 percent of the federal poverty guidelines[63]—the programs no longer align in states with BBCE policies that have raised the SNAP gross income limit. In the 27 states with BBCE gross income limits between 160 and 200 percent of the federal poverty guidelines, children in categorically eligible households may receive free school meals when, under traditional federal rules, they would not qualify for free meal assistance.[64] In short, through their BBCE policies, some states have effectively increased the income eligibility limits for two key federal nutrition assistance programs.

Inequities in Reporting Requirements

In states that have adopted BBCE, requirements for reporting changes in household income or household size can vary, resulting in unequal treatment of households. Under simplified reporting rules adopted by nearly all states,[65] households are required to report changes in income between scheduled reporting periods only if income exceeds the federal SNAP gross income limit—130 percent of the federal poverty guidelines. Because of BBCE, however, 27 states have, in effect, changed their SNAP gross income limit to levels greater than 130 percent. USDA issued SNAP guidance on change reporting requirements clarifying that, in states with simplified reporting, categorically eligible households with gross incomes over 130 percent of the federal poverty guidelines at the time of certification have no federal SNAP reporting requirements until they recertify or file a periodic report.[66] While guidance further indicates that states may choose to require these households to report when their gross income exceeds the income limit of the TANF program that confers

---

[63] 42 U.S.C. § 1758(b)(1)(A).

[64] Under school meals rules, children in families with gross household incomes between 130 and 185 percent of the federal poverty guidelines, while not eligible for free meals, are eligible to receive reduced price meals. 42 U.S.C. § 1758(b)(1)(A).

[65] As of November 2010, all states, except California and Wyoming, used simplified reporting for at least some SNAP households.

[66] One of the recent documents that provides this guidance is the Memo to Regional Directors, "Categorical Eligibility Questions and Answers," signed by the Director of the Program Development Division, FNS, USDA. January 26, 2010.

categorical eligibility, they are not required to do so. Two states we visited do not require households with incomes above 130 percent of the poverty guidelines to report changes in income between reporting periods. This results in lower-income SNAP households having a greater reporting burden than higher income SNAP households in order to retain their benefits.

While USDA has issued guidance to states in this area, its guidance relies on TANF reporting requirements that do not exist. USDA officials told us that TANF rules require categorically eligible SNAP households to report to TANF when their incomes exceed the income limit of the TANF service used to confer BBCE. However, because BBCE households are often authorized to receive a TANF-funded service through a brochure or toll-free telephone number given to them by a SNAP office, they may not be aware of any related TANF reporting requirements. Further, as we have previously reported, state TANF agencies are not required to collect data on many recipients of TANF-funded services, which include BBCE households.[67] Accordingly, a state TANF agency would not seek information on these households' income changes in order to share that information with the SNAP agency.

Conclusions

In response to the recent economic downturn and prolonged recovery, the Supplemental Nutrition Assistance Program has grown to provide unprecedented numbers of low-income households with benefits for food assistance. While the substantial increases in SNAP participation led to concerns that the large number of states adopting BBCE policies in recent years may have been a driver of those increases, these policies have had only a modest impact on program participation. Further, SNAP generally continues to serve households with the same types of characteristics it always has, and is intended to.

As federal and state governments face mounting fiscal pressures and confront limited resources, ensuring the integrity of SNAP and other programs spending public dollars is critical. While USDA touted BBCE as a way to improve program integrity and administrative efficiency, state adoption of BBCE has created unintended consequences that may

[67]GAO, *Temporary Assistance for Needy Families: Implications of Caseload and Program Changes for Families and Program Monitoring*, GAO-10-815T (Washington, D.C.: Sept. 21, 2010).

weaken both SNAP and related programs' integrity and introduce inequities. First, because gaps exist in USDA's review of states' procedures for implementing BBCE, some states are deeming households eligible under BBCE without following the required steps to do so. In addition, it is not known whether states are following the funding requirements associated with these policies. Second, because USDA's guidance clarifying children's eligibility for free school meals when their families receive $0 in SNAP benefits—an outcome likely more common because of BBCE—has not reached all states, school meal programs are vulnerable to overpayments and abuse. Finally, USDA's guidance on SNAP reporting requirements has resulted in lower-income households eligible under federal SNAP rules having to do more to retain their benefits than higher-income SNAP households eligible solely because of states' BBCE policies.

While these unintended consequences of BBCE on SNAP program integrity are potentially significant, they may also be easily addressed by those overseeing and administering the program. At a time when the economy has left more in need of assistance, SNAP continues to help low-income households obtain adequate nutrition. As a result, any changes to BBCE should carefully weigh the potential benefits and costs, which at this time include the increased burden on state and local staff who are already stretched thin as a result of decreased budgets and staff resources.

Recommendations for Executive Action

To improve SNAP program integrity and oversight, we are recommending that the Secretary of Agriculture require FNS to take several actions:

- Review state procedures for implementing BBCE, specifically those in place for providing the relevant TANF-funded service to all SNAP applicants deemed eligible under BBCE, as well as ensuring the relevant service is funded with TANF dollars.
- Disseminate the agency's October 2011 guidance clarifying that children in households certified as eligible for $0 in SNAP benefits should not be directly certified to receive free school meals directly to state agencies administering SNAP.
- Revisit agency guidance on change reporting requirements to ensure that all households, including those deemed eligible under BBCE with incomes above the federal gross income limit, are treated equitably.

Agency Comments and Our Evaluation

We provided a draft of this report to USDA for review and comment. On July 16, 2012, the Associate Administrator for SNAP and other FNS officials provided us with the agency's oral comments. Officials stated that they were in general agreement with the findings and recommendations presented in the report and offered technical comments that we have incorporated as appropriate. Officials also discussed the positive impacts BBCE has had on SNAP, including state administrative relief and cost savings, and emphasized our finding that BBCE policies have generally not changed the characteristics of SNAP households. As a result, the program continues to serve those it is intended to. Officials also noted their agreement with our conclusion that BBCE's benefits should be considered when assessing changes to these policies. Concerning our finding on the percentage of SNAP households with incomes over the federal limits that had payment errors, officials noted that these households may be more likely to have benefit errors than other SNAP households because they have greater earned income and deductions—factors that have been found to increase the likelihood of errors. We agree, and our findings on the characteristics of this sub-group of households support that conclusion. Further, officials suggested that the total amount of benefit dollars provided in error to this sub-group of households is likely relatively small because the average monthly benefit provided to these households is much smaller than the average benefit provided to all other SNAP households. Because of this, officials believe that errors in these households impact the overall SNAP payment error rate to a small extent, which is supported by the fact that the program's error rate has been relatively constant in recent years while the number of states with BBCE has increased. While we agree that it is likely that the total amount of benefit dollars provided in error to this sub-group of households is relatively small, we did not develop such an estimate during our analysis of the SNAP quality control data.

As agreed with your offices, unless you publicly announce the contents of this report earlier, we plan no further distribution of it until 30 days from the report date. At that time, we will send copies of this report to the appropriate congressional committees, the Secretary of Agriculture, and other interested parties. In addition, this report will be available at no charge on GAO's website at http://www.gao.gov.

If you or your staff have any questions concerning this report, please contact me at (202) 512-7215 or brownke@gao.gov. Contact points for our Offices of Congressional Relations and Public Affairs may be found on the last page of this report. GAO staff who made key contributions to this report are listed in appendix III.

Kay C. Brown

Kay E. Brown
Director, Education, Workforce, and Income Security Issues

Appendix I: Objectives, Scope, and Methodology

U.S. Department of Agriculture (USDA) Data Analysis

Quality Control Data

To determine the prevalence and characteristics of households deemed eligible under states' broad-based categorical eligibility (BBCE) policies that had incomes over the federal Supplemental Nutrition Assistance Program (SNAP) eligibility limits in fiscal years 2008 and 2010, we analyzed the Food and Nutrition Service's (FNS) quality control (QC) system data of active SNAP cases.[1] Per federal SNAP requirements, state officials draw monthly random samples of SNAP cases and review them to determine the extent to which households received benefits to which they were entitled. FNS officials in its regional offices and headquarters perform a secondary review of a sub-set of each state's sample of cases. The weighted analyses of the QC data produce nationally representative results.

To identify which households were deemed eligible under BBCE, and the sub-set of BBCE households that had incomes over the federal SNAP eligibility limits, we took several steps. First, we identified which states had BBCE policies in place in fiscal years 2008 and 2010 using an FNS compilation of BBCE policy implementation dates. Based on our discussions with FNS officials, Mathematica Policy Research, Inc. staff,[2] and state and local staff we spoke to during our five site visits, we assumed that once BBCE was enacted by a state, it was used as the default SNAP eligibility policy. Therefore, in states with BBCE policies in the fiscal year analyzed, we considered BBCE households to be those denoted in the QC data as categorically eligible in which all members did not receive cash assistance from another means-tested program. From this group, we determined the sub-set of BBCE households that had incomes over the federal SNAP eligibility limits.

We obtained the QC data directly from the QC database, which is made available to the public via Mathematica Policy Research, Inc.'s Web site.

---

[1] We reviewed information on SNAP in the 50 states; Washington, D.C.; Guam; and the Virgin Islands. We use "states" throughout the report to refer to this group.

[2] FNS contracts with Mathematica Policy Research, Inc. to maintain the SNAP QC data.

To analyze the data, we reviewed the technical user's manual for both the 2008 and 2010 QC public release data sets and evaluated the sampling methodology used to produce the data. We also reviewed the documentation for the internal review and coding process that FNS follows to prepare the QC data. Further, we checked the variables used in our analysis for out-of-range values or outliers. To produce weighted frequencies, weighted percents, and weighted dollar estimates for QC variables at the state and national level, we used the household weight variable provided in the public release QC data set. Because the records in the SNAP QC data are from a random sample, data analysis results are weighted estimates for a population of eligible households and thus are subject to sampling errors associated with samples of this size and type. The QC sample is only one of a large number of samples that states might have drawn. As each sample could have provided different estimates, we expressed our confidence in the precision of our QC data estimates as a 95 percent confidence interval (e.g., plus or minus 10 percentage points). To produce 95 percent confidence intervals around our weighted estimates, we used a statistical software package and an appropriate variance estimation method suitable for the sample design of the QC data. (Appendix II provides the estimates and 95 percent confidence intervals for the data we present in the body of this report.)

Through our analysis of the QC data, a review of the technical documentation, and interviews with FNS officials and Mathematica statisticians, we determined that the QC public release data were sufficiently reliable for the purposes of our audit.

In addition to conducting our own analysis of the QC data, we reviewed national-level data on SNAP payment error rates—the percentage of SNAP benefits paid in error—available from FNS for fiscal years 2000 to 2010. We also reviewed the primary sources of payment errors from 2000-2010 to help identify the extent to which payment errors were attributable to assets or another source.

Other SNAP Data

In addition to the QC data, we reviewed other data on SNAP participation and costs from USDA. Specifically, we analyzed data on average monthly SNAP participation in recent years obtained from USDA reports. In addition, we obtained data on total benefit costs and the average monthly SNAP benefits per household from USDA's Web site and the annual SNAP State Activity Reports for fiscal years 2001-2011, as well as data on the proportion of households receiving the maximum SNAP benefit from the annual Characteristics of SNAP Households reports for fiscal years 2001-2010. To assess administrative costs, we obtained data on federal and state outlays and obligations for fiscal years 2001-2010 from USDA's National Data Bank. These data are annually reported by states on the Standard Form 269 in specific cost categories designated by USDA. In addition, we obtained data on state expenditures of the federal Recovery Act funds provided for state administrative expenses in fiscal years 2009 and 2010, as well as the related funds provided through the Department of Defense Appropriations Act, 2010.

Site Visits

To better understand the effects of state BBCE policies on SNAP, as well as other factors impacting SNAP, we conducted site visits to 5 states and 18 local offices responsible for administering SNAP in those states, during January and February 2012. The states and localities we visited were Arizona—Maricopa, Pima, and Pinal counties; Illinois—Cook and Lake counties; North Carolina—Cabarrus, Gaston, Lincoln, and Mecklenburg counties; South Carolina—Greenville, Laurens, and Pickens counties; and Wisconsin—Kenosha, Milwaukee, and Racine counties. We selected these states because they varied in their BBCE adoption dates, in the characteristics of their BBCE policies, and in their geographic locations. States selected also had relatively large SNAP caseloads and generally high proportions of their SNAP households deemed eligible under BBCE policies.

In each state, we interviewed state officials responsible for administering SNAP, as well as local SNAP administrators and caseworkers at three or four local offices. The local offices we visited ranged from urban to rural areas. During the interviews we collected information about the state's BBCE policy and its application. In addition, we collected information about recent trends in SNAP participation, benefit amounts, administrative workload, and program errors, as well as BBCE's impact on each. We also collected information on other economic and non-economic factors that have impacted SNAP. Also, at each local office we observed the office's general process for serving SNAP applicants, including the forms, documents, and technological systems used, and we gathered information on how BBCE was applied during the process. Lastly, we conducted interviews with federal officials at the USDA regional office associated with each state in order to discuss their role in the oversight of SNAP. We cannot generalize our findings beyond the states and localities we visited.

Table 4: SNAP Households That Would Not Have Been Eligible for the Program without BBCE because Their Incomes Were over Federal Limits, in Fiscal Year 2010

	Estimate	95 percent confidence interval
SNAP households deemed eligible under BBCE with incomes over federal limits as a percentage of all SNAP households	2.6%	2.4% - 2.8%
SNAP households deemed eligible under BBCE with incomes over federal limits	473,381	438,088 - 508,675
All SNAP households	18,369,228	18,332,348 - 18,406,108
SNAP households deemed eligible under BBCE with incomes over federal limits as a percentage of SNAP households in states with BBCE policies that increased the gross income limit	4.8%	4.4% - 5.2%
SNAP households deemed eligible under BBCE with incomes over federal limits in states with BBCE policies that increased the gross income limit	405,927	374,464 - 437,390
All SNAP households in states with BBCE policies that increased the gross income limit	8,423,615	8,398,837 - 8,448,393
Average total income of SNAP households deemed eligible under BBCE with incomes over federal limits	$1,965	$1,919 - $2,010
Average total income of SNAP households deemed eligible under BBCE with incomes over federal limits as a percentage of the federal poverty guidelines	151%	149% - 153%

Source: GAO analysis of USDA's SNAP quality control data.

Table 5: Characteristics of Specified Groups of SNAP Households, in Fiscal Year 2010

	Estimate	95 percent confidence interval
SNAP households with at least one child as a percentage of:		
• SNAP households deemed eligible under BBCE with incomes over federal limits	56.3%	52.5% - 60.1%
• all other SNAP households	48.5%	47.9% - 49.1%
SNAP households with a single female as the head as a percentage of:		
• SNAP households deemed eligible under BBCE with incomes over federal limits	30.7%	27.2% - 34.2%
• all other SNAP households	25.8%	25.3% - 26.3%

	Estimate	95 percent confidence interval
SNAP households with at least one member receiving Social Security benefits as a percentage of:		
• SNAP households deemed eligible under BBCE with incomes over federal limits	27.8%	24.3% - 31.4%
• all other SNAP households	21.2%	20.8% - 21.7%
Average amount of Social Security benefits received by:		
• SNAP households deemed eligible under BBCE with incomes over federal limits	$340	$293 - $388
• all other SNAP households	$155	$151 - $159
SNAP households with at least one member with unearned income as a percentage of:		
• SNAP households deemed eligible under BBCE with incomes over federal limits	60.0%	56.3% - 63.7%
• all other SNAP households	60.3%	59.7% - 60.9%
SNAP households with at least one member with earned income as a percentage of:		
• SNAP households deemed eligible under BBCE with incomes over federal limits	65.9%	62.2% - 69.5%
• all other SNAP households	29.0%	28.4% - 29.5%
SNAP households with at least one member receiving Unemployment Insurance benefits as a percentage of:		
• SNAP households deemed eligible under BBCE with incomes over federal limits	18.6%	15.6% - 21.6%
• all other SNAP households	6.4%	6.1% - 6.7%
Average amount of Unemployment Insurance benefits received by:		
• SNAP households deemed eligible under BBCE with incomes over federal limits	$223	$185 - $262
• all other SNAP households	$55	$52 - $58

Source: GAO analysis of USDA's SNAP quality control data.

Table 6: Benefits Provided to SNAP Households That Would Not Have Been Eligible for the Program without BBCE because Their Incomes were over Federal Limits, per Month in Fiscal Year 2010

	Estimate	95 percent confidence interval
SNAP benefits provided to households deemed eligible under BBCE with incomes over federal limits as a percentage of all SNAP benefits	0.7%	0.6% - 0.8%
SNAP benefits provided to households deemed eligible under BBCE with incomes over federal limits	$38,333,145	33,972,894 – 42,693,395
Total amount of benefits provided to all SNAP households	$5,273,937,192	5,227,633,694 – 5,320,240,691
SNAP benefits provided to households deemed eligible under BBCE with incomes over federal limits as a percentage of all SNAP benefits in states with BBCE policies that increased the gross income limit	1.5%	1.3% - 1.6%
SNAP benefits provided to households deemed eligible under BBCE with incomes over federal limits in states with BBCE policies that increased the gross income limit	$33,987,767	$30,127,143 - $37,848,392
Total amount of benefits provided to all SNAP households in states with BBCE policies that increased the gross income limit	$2,308,594,258	$2,277,254,048 - $2,339,934,469

Source: GAO analysis of USDA's SNAP quality control data.

Table 7: Benefits Received by Specified Groups of SNAP Households, in Fiscal Year 2010

	Estimate	95 Percent Confidence Interval
Average monthly SNAP benefit received by:		
• SNAP households deemed eligible under BBCE with incomes over federal limits	$81	$74 - $88
• all other SNAP households	$293	$290 - 295
SNAP households receiving the minimum benefit as a percentage of:		
• SNAP households deemed eligible under BBCE with incomes over federal limits	44.3%	40.3% - 48.1%
• all other SNAP households	2.7%	2.5% - 2.9%

Source: GAO analysis of USDA's SNAP quality control data.

Table 8: Estimated Percent of Specified Groups of SNAP Households Receiving Deductions and the Estimated Average Amount of the Deduction in Fiscal Year 2010

	Estimate	95 Percent Confidence Interval
SNAP households receiving child support deduction as a percentage of:		
• SNAP households deemed eligible under BBCE with incomes over federal limits	6.7%	4.6% - 8.9%
• all other SNAP households	1.9%	1.7% - 2.0%
Average amount of child support deduction received by:		
• SNAP households deemed eligible under BBCE with incomes over federal limits	$20	$13 - $27
• all other SNAP households	$4	$4 - $5
SNAP households receiving dependent care deduction as a percentage of:		
• SNAP households deemed eligible under BBCE with incomes over federal limits	14.3%	11.6% - 17.0%
• all other SNAP households	3.5%	3.3% - 3.7%
Average amount of dependent care deduction received by:		
• SNAP households deemed eligible under BBCE with incomes over federal limits	$50	$37 - $62
• all other SNAP households	$8	$7 - $8
SNAP households receiving earned income deduction as a percentage of:		
• SNAP households deemed eligible under BBCE with incomes over federal limits	65.9%	62.2% - 69.5%
• all other SNAP households	28.9%	28.4% - 29.5%
Average amount of earned income deduction received by:		
• SNAP households deemed eligible under BBCE with incomes over federal limits	$243	$227 - $260
• all other SNAP households	$57	$56 - $59
SNAP households receiving medical deduction as a percentage of:		
• SNAP households deemed eligible under BBCE with incomes over federal limits	13.0%	10.3% - 15.8%
• all other SNAP households	3.5%	3.3% - 3.8%
Average amount of medical deduction received by:		
• SNAP households deemed eligible under BBCE with incomes over federal limits	$19	$14 - $25
• all other SNAP households	$5	$5 - $6

	Estimate	95 Percent Confidence Interval
SNAP households receiving excess shelter deduction as a percentage of:		
• SNAP households deemed eligible under BBCE with incomes over federal limits	72.2%	68.7% - 75.6%
• all other SNAP households	70.5%	70.0% - 71.1%
Average amount of excess shelter deduction received by:		
• SNAP households deemed eligible under BBCE with incomes over federal limits	$220	$205 - $235
• all other SNAP households	$265	$263 - $268

Source: GAO analysis of USDA's SNAP quality control data.

Appendix III: GAO Contacts and Staff Acknowledgments

GAO Contact	Kay E. Brown, (202) 512-7215 or brownke@gao.gov
Staff Acknowledgments	Kathy Larin (Assistant Director), Rachel Frisk (Analyst-in-Charge), Avani Locke, and David Perkins made significant contributions to all aspects of this report. Also contributing to this report were Carl Barden, Marquita Campbell, Susannah Compton, Heather Dunahoo, Greg Kutz, Jean McSween, Mimi Nguyen, Susan Offutt, Rhiannon Patterson, Kathy Peyman, Almeta Spencer, Craig Winslow, and Jill Yost.

Related GAO Products

State and Local Governments: Knowledge of Past Recessions Can Inform Future Federal Fiscal Assistance. GAO-11-401. Washington, D.C.: March 31, 2011.

Temporary Assistance for Needy Families: Implications of Caseload and Program Changes for Families and Program Monitoring. GAO-10-815T. Washington, D.C.: September 21, 2010.

Supplemental Nutrition Assistance Program: Payment Errors and Trafficking Have Declined, but Challenges Remain. GAO-10-956T. Washington, D.C.: July 28, 2010.

Domestic Food Assistance: Complex System Benefits Millions, but Additional Efforts Could Address Potential Inefficiency and Overlap among Smaller Programs. GAO-10-346. Washington, D.C.: April 15, 2010.

Food Stamp Program: FNS Could Improve Guidance and Monitoring to Help Ensure Appropriate Use of Noncash Categorical Eligibility. GAO-07-465. Washington, D.C.: March 28, 2007.

Human Service Programs: Demonstration Projects Could Identify Ways to Simplify Policies and Facilitate Technology Enhancements to Reduce Administrative Costs. GAO-06-942. Washington, D.C.: September 19, 2006.

Food Stamp Program: States Have Made Progress Reducing Payment Errors, and Further Challenges Remain. GAO-05-245. Washington, D.C.: May 5, 2005.

Food Stamp Program: Farm Bill Options Ease Administrative Burden, but Opportunities Exist to Streamline Participant Reporting Rules among Programs. GAO-04-916. Washington, D.C.: September 16, 2004.

Food Stamp Program: Steps Have Been Taken to Increase Participation of Working Families, but Better Tracking of Efforts Is Needed. GAO-04-346. Washington, D.C.: March 5, 2004.

Food Stamp Program: States' Use of Options and Waivers to Improve Program Administration and Promote Access. GAO-02-409. Washington, D.C.: February 22, 2002.

Means-Tested Programs: Determining Financial Eligibility Is Cumbersome and Can Be Simplified. GAO-02-58. Washington, D.C.: November 2, 2001.

Food Stamp Program: States Seek to Reduce Payment Errors and Program Complexity. GAO-01-272. Washington, D.C.: January 19, 2001.